A Creator's Guide to
Stopping Self-Harm

Maggie Parr ―――――

The Creator's Guide to Stopping Self-Harm by Maggie Parr
©2024, Maggie Parr
Published by Obedon Books, Petaluma, CA

"Intrusion" By Denise Levertov, from Poems 1968-72, copyright ©1971 by Denise Levertov. Reprinted by permission of New Directions Publishing Corp.

Excerpt from "The Niagara River" from The Niagara River copyright © 2005 by Kay Ryan. Used with permission.

"Hope is the Thing With Feathers" by Emily Dickenson, from The Poems of Emily Dickinson: Reading Edition, edited by Ralph W. Franklin, Cambridge, Mass.: The Belknap Press of Harvard University Press, Copyright © 1998, 1999 by the President and Fellows of Harvard College. Copyright © 1951, 1955, 1979, 1983 by the President and Fellows of Harvard College.

All rights reserved. No part of this publication may be reproduced, distributed, or transmitted in any form or by any means, including photocopying, recording, or other electronic or mechanical methods, without prior written permission of the author, except in the case of brief quotations embodied in critical reviews and certain other noncommercial uses permitted by copyright law.

The author does not make any guarantees about the results of the information given in this book. Educational and informational resources contained within these pages are intended to help the reader succeed in stopping self-harm. Readers' ultimate success or failure will be the result of their own efforts, particular situations, and innumerable other circumstances beyond the author's knowledge and control. The resources in this book are provided for informational purposes only and should not be used to replace the specialized training and professional judgment of a health care or mental health care professional.

For more information, email inquire@obedonpress.com.

ISBN: 979-8-9910743-0-8 (paperback)
ISBN: 979-8-9910743-1-5 (ebook)
ISBN: 979-8-9910743-2-2 (audiobook)

If you would like to access examples of the exercises in this book, go to www.stoppingselfharm.com/guide to download the free guide. It contains images, visualizations, templates, and additional resources. For deeper work, you can also sign up for an interactive online course based on the topics in this book, using creativity to heal from self-injury and trauma.

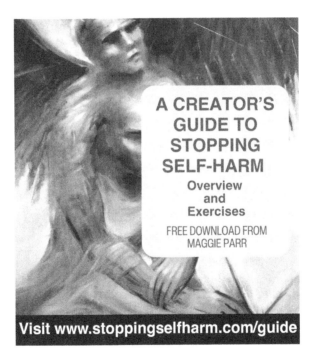

If you would like to view Maggie Parr's artwork or learn more about her services as teacher and creative coach, visit www.maggieparr.com.

For my brother Andy, who started in the darkness with me, but left before he could find his way out.

TABLE OF CONTENTS

Chapter One: Overview 1

Chapter Two: Why Creativity? 17

Chapter Three: Prepare for the Journey 45

Chapter Four: The Child and the Spirit Guide 68

Chapter Five: Faith in the Darkness 95

Chapter Six: Hope is the Glue 124

Chapter Seven: Love the Work 144

Chapter Eight: Allowing Grace 173

Chapter Nine: Back to the Beginning 194

Before You Begin:

Self-harming is a serious concern and should not be taken lightly. This book is a creative guide written by someone who recovered from the behavior—but only with years of work with a qualified therapist and psychiatrist. Maggie Parr is not a professional counselor. If you are considering embarking on your own journey of healing, use this book as an adjunct to therapy, not as a replacement.

If you have suicidal thoughts or feelings, seek help immediately by calling 988, or go to your nearest emergency room.

Intrusion

After I had cut off my hands and grown new ones

something my former hands had longed for came and asked to be rocked.

After my plucked out eyes had withered, and new ones grown

something my former eyes had wept for

came asking to be pitied.

—Denise Levertov

CHAPTER ONE

OVERVIEW

If you've picked up this book, you've either had experience with self-injury, or you know someone who does. Perhaps you're a clinician trying to help a client. Or a parent who is worried about your child's behaviors.

The first thing I want to assure you is that *you are not alone*. I struggled with cutting and self-harming behaviors for most of my life. If I wasn't actually doing it, I was trying not to. When I managed to stop in my thirties, it was because I'd built an elaborate defense around me to protect against triggers; and when that fell apart, the self-injury returned with a vengeance. I was frightened of my lack of control, and desperate for help.

But there wasn't much out there for a forty-four-year-old, even in 2012. Most people still associate self-injury with middle-class, white, teenage girls. Although it is true that about 17 percent of teenagers self-harm, according to the American Psychological Association (APA), approximately 35 percent of those are male, a statistic which is likely underreported. Also, about 1.3 percent of children between 5–10 self-injure, as do 5–6 percent of adults. Demographic research holds this to be true regardless of race/

ethnic identity or socioeconomic status.[1] If those statistics are applied to current population figures, over fourteen *million* people are self-harming in the United States alone.

It's not just in the U.S., either. A recent meta-analysis of the prevalence of self-injury behaviors during the COVID-19 pandemic across America, Europe, Asia, and Oceana showed an average of 14.6 percent in ages ranging from adolescence up to 60 years of age.[2]

In fact, it's not even limited to our species. Other animals do it, too, if they're miserable and trapped in places like medical labs. To name just one example, the Animal Welfare Institute reported that "Approximately 10% of captive, individually-housed monkeys engage in the disturbing phenomenon of self-injurious behavior (SIB)."[3]

The second thing to know is that it's not some weird defect or unexplainable phenomenon. In humans, the behavior is often associated with childhood sexual abuse, but that's not the only causal factor. Studies show that children who experience bullying are more likely to self-injure, as do LGBTQ+ populations, probably because of the lack of acceptance from peers and families. Anecdotally, I've noticed in myself and others who self-harm that we experienced confusing messages growing up, such as a disconnect between spoken words and actions, or a pressure to conform.

---

[1] American Psychological Association, *Monitor on Psychology*, Vol. 46, No. 47, July/August 2015, https://www.apa.org/monitor/2015/07-08/who-self-injures.

[2] Juan Cheng, Di Wang, Lu Wang, Haiou Zou, Yuanhua Qu, "Global Prevalence of Self-Harm during the Covid-19 pandemic: a systematic review and meta-analysis," *BMC Psychol.*, 2023, 11:149, https://www.ncbi.nlm.nih.gov/pmc/articles/PMC10160734/.

[3] Viktor Reinhardt and Matt Rossell, "Self-Biting in Caged Macaques: Cause, Effect, and Treatment, n.d., https://awionline.org/content/self-biting-caged-macaques-cause-effect-and-treatment#:~:text=Injurious%20self%2Dbiting%20is%20one,%2Dinjurious%20behavior%20(SIB).

OVERVIEW

Whatever the cause, somewhere along the way, we lost our ability to express ourselves. Self-injury became a kind of voice on the skin. It's a maladaptive coping mechanism—a natural response to overwhelming emotions. When it feels like there's no other way out, what we still have control over is our bodies—and self-inflicted pain can actually feel soothing. We cut and burn our skin, tear out hair, break bones, force ourselves to vomit, and any number of behaviors to try and control what's going on inside.

The problem is, once we pick up these habits, they're hard to stop. They become addictive. Chemical reactions take place beyond our conscious thought, and we repeat the cycle over and over again. We lose control over what started as a way to gain control. If the self-harming behavior is extreme or obvious, it scares our loved ones—and they urge us to stop, which only makes it harder.

Then there's the issue of fear. What will happen to me if I let go of this self-soothing behavior that scares people? "Fear" is too soft a word—it's more like *terror*. There's a reason we picked up this behavior—to protect our psyches from harm—so to just drop it without new coping mechanisms can be more damaging than helpful.

And what do we do with all those unbearable *feelings*? Self-harming regulates the internal chaos. It brings relief, a sense of calm. Without it, anger blooms into rage, fear becomes terror, sadness sinks into despair without end.

Psychologists, doctors, and scientists have been studying, researching, analyzing, and categorizing these behaviors for decades. They used to assume that self-injury was an attention-seeking behavior, usually a symptom of Borderline Personality Disorder (BPD). But newer studies have shown that most who self-harm go to great lengths to hide it. It is now listed in the current Diagnostic and Statistical Manual of Mental Disorders (DSM-5) as non-suicidal self-injury, or NSSI, and is named as one of the "Conditions for Further Study." As E. David Klonsky et al. define it, "NSSI refers to the intentional destruction of one's own body tissue without suicidal intent and for purposes not socially sanctioned. Common examples include cutting, burning, scratching, and banging or hitting, and most people who self-injure have used multiple methods."[4]

Although not considered a suicidal gesture, the frequency of NSSI is strongly correlated with subsequent suicide attempts. NSSI often occurs alongside eating disorders, substance abuse, and, not surprisingly, anxiety and/or depression. Emotional dysregulation and dissociation are common in all of the various self-harming habits. Each has its own official diagnosis—NSSI, bulimia nervosa or purging disorder, trichotillomania, deliberate self-poisoning (DSP), substance abuse disorder, etc. Each comes with a range of recommended modalities and medications. But none address the person as a whole, or the underlying reasons for the need to self-harm in the first place.

The officially sanctioned approaches are limited at best and, at their worst, can be further damaging. As the psychologist Richard C. Schwartz stated, "giving a troubled person a psychiatric diagnosis and seeing that as the sole or main cause of their symptoms [is] unnecessarily limiting, pathologizing, and could become self-reinforcing."[5]

Many psychiatrists and psychologists, frustrated by the lack of official direction, have moved beyond current protocols to

---

[4] E. David Klonsky, PhD, Sarah E. Victor, MA, and Boaz Y. Saffer, BA, "Non-Suicidal Self-Injury: What We Know, and What We Need to Know," *Can J Psychiatry* (November 2014), 565-68, https://www.ncbi.nlm.nih.gov/pmc/articles/PMC4244874/.

[5] Richard Schwartz, *No Bad Parts: Healing Trauma and Restoring Wholeness with the Internal Family Systems Model* (Sounds True, 2021, Kindle edition), 58.

develop their own approaches through trial and error. Sometimes, they create new modalities (complete with trademarks, books, and subsequent training programs); sometimes, they simply listen to their clients' intuition and guide them toward healing.

I was fortunate to encounter one of those latter kinds of therapists. My desperate search for help in my forties led me to her office. She'd received training in various methods but didn't align herself with specific modalities. Instead, she brought all of her knowledge and instinct into every session—which she described as "two people in a room." With her help, I was finally able to look at *why* I'd self-harmed—and embrace what (and who) I found in the process. I realized how much creativity and imagination had guided my journey through my lifelong quest to find relief from internal pain.

This book is a culmination of what I discovered. It's meant to offer suggestions to others who want to forge their own healing, using the tools available within themselves. Psychology and psychiatry offer invaluable tools—but the only person who can do the hard work of change is the one who wants to heal.

And that is something I know how to do.

The third important truth I want to convey through this book is that people *can* stop self-injury—through creativity, compassion, and guidance. I did it, and I've been free from any urges since 2016. I've also helped many others find self-love through visualizations, creative exercises, and encouragement.

In the process of healing from self-harm, we not only resolve past traumas, but we find the thing we've been looking for all along: our truest self.

My Experience

I was fourteen when I first revealed my wounds to the psychology intern at the local counseling clinic. By that point, I'd been cutting my forehead with a razor blade for two years. That counselor later told me that neither she nor her supervisor had seen the behavior before. It was 1981, and the American Psychiatric Association had only just created the diagnosis of Post-Traumatic Stress Disorder (PTSD), thanks to the lobbying efforts of veterans and the doctors who worked with them. The field of psychology was still years away from acknowledging how childhood abuse and trauma play a role in mental health struggles.

I was a textbook case. My father sexually abused both my brother and me, while my mother dissociated and denied what was happening. I first self-harmed at four, when I scratched my arm repeatedly with a safety pin. As I got older, I stabbed my palms with pencils and banged my head against the corners of doors. I fought other kids, broke rules, stole from the local store, and caused mayhem. Today, teachers would be able to identify my behaviors and call the authorities, but back then, no one knew what to do with a troubled child who didn't get along well with others. Instead, I was paddled, locked in a closet, taken to the principal's office, or sent home from school. Occasionally, a teacher took pity on me and offered extra attention and nurturing; others vented their frustration on me, compounding my reactiveness. I can mark the years where I had a kind and empathetic teacher by my grades.

Dad stopped abusing me when I was ten. He also became distant and started drinking more. By the time I was twelve, the loneliness and confusing feelings were unbearable. I picked up the razor blades at the same time that I began self-poisoning through pills. My parents were too consumed with their own struggles to notice. Dad spiraled into full-blown alcoholism, and my stressed-out mother could barely take care of herself, let alone us. But when I was fourteen, she asked if I wanted to see her counselor, and I accepted. I was finally able to tell someone what I was doing and ask for help. That started me on a lifelong search for answers.

It was a race to outsmart the pain. As I stumbled through adolescence, my arsenal of coping mechanisms expanded into alcoholism, substance abuse, bulimia, promiscuity, and suicide attempts. Creativity and artmaking became my first line of defense as I figured out ways to stay alive. Over-achievement helped, although it often veered into workaholism. Team sports taught me discipline and agency but led to an exercising addiction that generated problems later.

In college and after, the search for relief led me to therapists, recovery groups, spiritual programs, workshops, modalities, and into relationships that I hoped would fix me (but never did). Getting sober at twenty-four built a foundation for my continuing recovery. It gave me a set of spiritual tools and a container to keep me safe. I stopped binging and purging and found periodic relief from cutting. Along the way, I read every book by Alice Miller, Judith Herman, Marilee Strong, Steven Levenkron, Peter Levine, Bessel van der Kolk, and more. Because they were written so much later than the onset of my self-injury, it was like reading about myself in hindsight. While researchers were doing their empirical studies and battling with the APA to modify the DSM's understanding of self-injury, I was living my life as best I could—building my career as an artist, scraping money together for therapy, and navigating relationships. I found pockets of real happiness amidst the ups and downs of depression.

I came of age just before the great medicating wave swept our country, so I was never given diagnoses or antidepressants—which is fortunate, because I would have been prescribed everything in the book. The over-medicating of my younger peers scared me, so I avoided getting psychiatric help for too long. During my twenties and thirties, I had a caring therapist who was with me through getting sober, dealing with the memories of abuse, and navigating my long-term relationship. To manage chronic depression, anxiety, and panic attacks, I cleaned up my diet and learned to meditate and do yoga. By thirty, I was able to quell the urges to self-harm.

Then in my mid-forties, I relapsed in cutting. My twenty-year relationship was in crisis, life's stressors were overwhelming, and I didn't have enough resources. I also started burning my arms with boiling water. My partner was appalled and frightened, and she pressured me to stop.

My old therapist was nearing retirement and I felt that our work together had run its course. So, I found a new therapist, one who would guide me back to myself. I was able to leave my relationship and start living on my own. I accepted medical advice and went on an antidepressant, which lifted my baseline of suicidal depression up into regular sadness, which I could then process in healthier ways. From there, I was able to go deeper into the core reasons for the self-injury.

And so, I faced what I'd been avoiding my whole life—the Cutter. That's what I called the part of myself that took over and injured my skin. Instead of hating it, trying to banish it from my psyche, I became curious about where it came from. By this time, it was the mid-teens of the 21st century, and trauma therapy had become an accepted modality. Techniques like Somatic Experiencing (SE) and Eye Movement Desensitization and Reprocessing (EMDR) addressed the mind-body connection. Yoga was being recommended to help patients and clients reconnect with their bodies. The humanistic approach to therapy had changed the

OVERVIEW

focus from hierarchical diagnoses and treatment to client-centered, whole-person modalities, fueled by compassion and connection.

One modality, Internal Family Systems (IFS), developed by Richard C. Schwartz, Ph.D., addressed what he'd learned through decades of working with bulimic clients. He discovered that we all have different parts of our psyches, but people who have experienced trauma have a harder time regulating these parts. The parts often battle each other, leading to distressing behaviors. By identifying and working with the fragmented selves, and recognizing that each plays an important role, a governing self can develop that not only heals the whole system, but also leads to spiritual growth.

I didn't discover IFS until after I wrote the first draft of this book, but I was amazed to read that what I'd found organically was being experienced all over the country. It affirmed for me that none of us do this alone. We're each part of a greater movement of healing, sharing, and evolving.

I came to these realizations slowly, painfully, over many years. Therapists guided me, recovery programs gave me tools, books led to insights; but it was my imagination and instinct for storytelling that created my path to healing. Writing and artmaking were as important to my recovery as therapy and medication. My spiritual connection provided the healing power that sutured old wounds. As I faced different challenges, new energies appeared, named themselves, and joined my inner pantheon. Finally, everything made sense inside. It didn't have to be quantifiably true—documented in double-blind experiments or listed in the DSM—it just had to ring true for *me*. That's all I was ever looking for—a self that I could *trust*, that would unite the disconnected parts and allow me to live a full life.

Along the way, I entered into a relationship that, for the first time, didn't mirror my family of origin. I learned what love really is, and I thrived within it. My chemistry calmed, my artwork mellowed, and the relentless suffering (and my focus on it) finally eased. And I discovered that all those years of struggle had hollowed out a huge well of love in my heart. My purpose shifted from finding relief from pain to helping others out of theirs.

This is the point at which this book begins—when I am finally able to say (and know) that I'm free from self-harming. Not because I've sworn off or buried it, but because I've gone to the core of what caused it and healed that wound. That's the journey I want to share with you so that you might chart your own path. The process of healing naturally awakens a deep desire to help others. I believe I've found a unique way into recovery that can be useful to artists and non-artists alike—not a list of labels that you must adopt to imitate what I experienced, but a suggested roadmap to guide you on your own journey.

About This Book

This book is for those who currently self-injure, as well as those who have in the past and want to learn more about why they did it. It's also for the clinicians who help them. It focuses on cutting and burning because that's what I struggled with most. But I also went through bulimia, drug and alcohol addiction, sex addiction, over-exercising, deliberate self-poisoning, and more—so the things I did to recover apply to more than one behavior. I found that by addressing the "dis-ease" at the heart of these addictions, each one resolved completely.

In all my research, I've found that books on self-harming fall into two categories: memoirs by those who recovered from a specific behavior, and analytical books by professionals who have either worked with clients or conducted empirical studies. All are valuable in their own ways. The memoirs are hard for me to get through because reading about someone else's self-injury triggers a bodily response that reminds me of my own trauma. I've gotten more help from the clinical studies—the information, guidance, and knowledge that I'm not alone—yet they didn't give me concrete ways to stop self-harming.

What I haven't found yet is the book I always wanted to read—an actual guide to stopping self-injury, written by someone who *did* it. That's what I've attempted to write, using all the experiences and lessons I learned along the way. The road to recovery took so much effort, time, and money that it was like getting a graduate degree. I know that kind of commitment isn't possible for everyone, so I feel compelled to share what I learned with others to ease the path toward recovery and reduce suffering wherever I can.

I know what it's like to be in the thick of self-harming and what it's like to be free of it. Therapy has been enormously helpful over the years, but sessions only last fifty minutes. I had to figure out how to get through the other 10,030 minutes in a week. I learned to manage my overwhelming feelings and urges, stop self-injuring, then sustain recovery over the long haul. I journeyed inward to find the parts of me that self-harmed, and finally listened to what they were trying to say. In the process, I found many unexpected gifts.

I realized that my art and creativity were valuable tools. If an urge overwhelmed me, I could cut into a painting instead of my skin. Writing and drawing gave voice to unspoken feelings and memories. When I let the Cutter create art, it gave my work powerful energy and changed my neural pathways. My lifelong body of work is an expression of that pilgrimage. It's taught me who I really am. As a result, I developed many creative exercises that might help others stop self-harming.

This book is a collection of those lessons. It might be described as *The Artist's Way* for readers of *The Body Keeps the Score*—a manual to harness innate creativity in the pathway to healing. Although it's geared toward the arts, and visual arts in particular, anyone can do these exercises. You don't have to be an artist. All you need is courage and an open mind.

This book is not a substitute for therapy; in fact, I highly recommend that if you want to do the exercises in this book, you work with a therapist to help you with the experiences that arise. I am *not* a doctor or counselor. I'm an artist who recovered from self-injury. Although I offer an overview of what professionals are doing to help people who self-injure, this account is based on my personal experiences and anecdotal observations. If you are trying to recover from self-harming, I encourage you to do your own research and see what works for you, to use this as a workbook—not as a one-size-fits-all prescription, but as a jumping-off point for your own self-directed path.

Although this isn't a stand-alone memoir, I will be telling parts of my story as they relate to the exercises in each chapter. I won't dwell on details of cutting or abuse. I don't want to activate anyone's trauma response. My intention is not to sensationalize, but to create a roadmap, based on my own journey, and to place markers on the path for others to follow. Ideally, it will guide readers along a route that leads to healing from self-harm and to sustaining recovery in the long term. At the bare minimum, I hope it provides inspiration.

I believe that once we travel to the core of what triggered the self-harming in the first place, and do our healing there, the need for the self-injury will naturally fall away. Willpower and hard work are required to wean ourselves from our addictions—but that, too, is easier once we have developed true compassion for ourselves.

OVERVIEW

This book is *not* a tool for those who want to "make" a loved one stop self-harming. I understand the desire to do so, as the behavior can be very frightening to those who see its aftermath. However, the decision to stop can only be made by the person who's doing it. Anything else is a form of control that will only backfire. Healing has to arise from within or else it won't last. Each person who struggles with self-injury needs to find their own agency, self-love, and self-actualization. There are many resources online to support those who have someone in their life who self-injures; I encourage you to do your own research and develop more compassion.

I want to emphasize again that no particular talent is needed to do the exercises in this book. As long as you have hands that work, you can do anything within these pages. I'll make a case for creativity as a therapeutic modality in the next chapter, and take you step by step through the process of drawing stick figures to completing works of art. But if you *really* don't like doing visual art, there are many other ways to express yourself creatively—and I will offer examples throughout.

We're all innately creative without adopting the title of "artist." Creativity is our human birthright, and I believe it's the key to unlocking the door to our highly personal, unique path toward recovery.

Chapter Breakdown

Each chapter is organized by a different theme or segment of the journey. I tie it to the history and attitudes in psychology and society, then I share my own personal experience. I offer different techniques and suggestions for grounding, containing, and connecting inside the mind and body. Then I share creative exercises that speak to each theme. They're accessible to anyone, artist or not. Even so, each chapter will end with one or more advanced activities for those who do identify as artists and want to deepen their work. Of course, anyone can try those exercises as well.

The visualizations in this book are taken directly from my personal experience. Since it's hard to read a meditation while *doing* it, I offer links to free online recordings of the meditations at www.stoppingselfharm.com. I've always had an active imagination, so it's easy for me to dip into it. Those who are struggling with active depression may have a harder time accessing vivid imagery and altered states. I have a cousin who achieved this through guided use of psychedelics, but I don't have experience with this, so I can't offer advice in this area. Although people who are open to creativity or versed in spiritual practices may have an easier time with meditation, anyone can learn how to go deep inside. It's another birthright—to explore our own interior.

Chapter two goes into more detail about why creativity is so important when it comes to healing from self-injury. Clinicians and researchers are finally measuring the positive benefits of artmaking on healing and neuroplasticity. The field of "Neuroarts" is rapidly growing into an accepted modality for healing. I'll share more of my story to show how I instinctively used creativity to heal old wounds and craft new stories—something I discovered long before science mirrored my findings. I'll prove to you that anyone can draw, starting with easy exercises that will show you how easy it is.

Chapters three and four are meant to prepare you for the journey inward. They give concrete techniques and creative exercises to ground yourself, create safety and containment, explore your inner world, make a spiritual connection, and practice creating art. I'll give more examples from my own life as well. By this point, you will see that my storytelling is more circular than linear, and the same experiences yield ever-deepening insights.

Chapters five through eight form the heart of this book. Here, I describe what it was like to meet my own Cutter and identify it as a dissociated part of me—a fragment of my traumatic childhood. Advocates of Internal Family Systems (IFS) may resonate with this part of the work. The activities in these chapters are designed to help you map your inner terrain to familiarize you with what your self-harming parts are trying to express. In sharing how the tapestry of my inner family wove together, I present a guide to your own re-weaving. Each chapter builds on the growth in the last so that the chaotic thoughts, emotions, and chemistry knit together as new avenues of expression are created.

The concluding chapter contains a message of encouragement. I know from my own experience and from observing others that permanent recovery from self-injury is not only possible, it's inevitable. Once we begin the work, all the forces of Creation will come to our aid.

But this isn't about simply stopping a behavior. The quest to discover what's causing it leads us to what we've been looking for all along. In creating our own path to healing, we gain the tools needed, the Self we've been looking for, and the resilience to face future challenges. The thing we thought was "broken" turns out to be our greatest strength.

Trust me. I've been through it and have come out the other side.

You are embarking on a quest for answers, a quest for the piece that's missing, for the healing that can only be found from deep within the wound. Don't be afraid—you've got this. You have so much to give, and it's time to reach in and discover what is really going on inside. The world needs you at your best, now more than ever.

"I pressed and dragged until I saw blood. Instantly my heartbeat receded from my ears, tucked itself calmly back into my rib cage, and my mind folded itself into a neat origami brain—clean, calm lines. The wild pitching was replaced by a thick stillness, the laceration a hot horizon, steadying and orienting me. It had come to me so easily, so naturally, and it had worked."

—Alice Carriére,
from *Everything/Nothing/Someone: A Memoir*

"...as a mouth on the flesh containedly expressing violence, self-mutilation provides the possibility of a new openness—of expressing what it is to be hurt and what it is to be aggressive—without either lying or becoming an abuser. This new possibility would not be the hand holding a razor blade which cuts across the skin, but breath being pushed across the larynx, shaped by mouth and tongue, into a spoken word."

—Janice McLane,
from *The Voice on the Skin: Self-Mutilation and Merleau-Ponty's Theory of Language*

CHAPTER TWO

WHY CREATIVITY?

The urge to harm oneself seems to defy reason. Why would anyone slice or burn their own skin? Or pull their hair out, or stick a finger down their throat, or do anything so obviously harmful to the body that holds them?

Because it's soothing. That's the truth, as counterintuitive as it seems. It makes us feel real. It brings a sense of power and agency. It opens a valve to release pressure so we can breathe again. It quiets the voices, organizes the chaos, and fills us with relief. No matter the shame or fear, we return to it again and again, seeking that comfort.

It's also inherently creative. Whatever initial experience led us to self-harm, we picked up the behavior in *response* to something. To keep ourselves intact in the face of painful stimuli. To express what was not allowed in words. To make sense of overwhelming emotions like fear, anger, confusion, and sadness. To solve an unsolvable problem. We choose a specific behavior, a specific part of the body to harm, and specific tools. Many of us engage in rituals—laying a towel on the floor, pulling out that special razor, playing music. Afterward, we might clean and bandage the wound or gently wash our faces. We feel calm, at peace, connected to ourselves and the world once again. We may even be in a state of transcendence.

Doesn't that sound like a spiritual experience?

If you take away the images of the body being harmed, it does look like a worshiper praying before their god. In a way, the act of self-harming is a plea: *Take away this pain, please. Restore me to wholeness, please.* It's our unique communion with a powerful, mysterious energy that brings us peace.

And so, if we want to stop the behavior, we need to find something just as powerful to replace it. Something creative, personal, and spiritual. Or, perhaps, just *creative*—because isn't the creative process inherently highly personal as well as spiritual?

Can we make art that's personal, expresses the nonverbal, and connects us to that energy of self-harming?

Artists and writers are often more comfortable with the idea of the Muse as an intermediary—a messenger of God/Spirit/Universal Intelligence that downloads information and inspiration into our art. It's a persistent archetype because it's universally experienced. Why else would a poet slave away at words for such a meager living? Or a painter hole up in their studio for years or a lifetime, toiling away at the canvas, searching for that perfect image? We're trying to feel that blessed relief that comes with getting it right. To gain that divine approval. To die knowing we did our best work in the service of our souls.

But artmaking doesn't belong only to the dedicated artist. It's a fundamental human practice, and it has measurable benefits on overall health.

Artists have known this for ages, but clinicians are finally beginning to prove this with science. Bessel van der Kolk put out the call in his 2015 book, *The Body Keeps the Score*—a thorough study of the effects of trauma on the body and mind—when he said:

> There are thousands of art, music, and dance therapists who do beautiful work with abused children, soldiers suffering from PTSD, incest victims, refugees, and torture survivors, and numerous accounts attest to the effectiveness of expressive therapies. However, at this point we know very little about how they work or about the specific aspects of traumatic stress they address, and it would present an enormous logistical and financial challenge to do the research necessary to establish their value scientifically.[6]

Enormously challenging, perhaps, but not impossible. Since then, many scientists and clinicians have attempted to quantify the benefits of arts-related treatment for trauma. Susan Magsamen and Ivy Ross assembled much of the research being done in the field of "Neuroarts" in their 2023 book, *Your Brain on Art*. In it, they cite study after study showing the positive neurological effects of art-making, dancing, acting, writing, playing music, attending events and museums, and even being in a culturally enriched environment. These practices rewire neural pathways, develop resiliency, foster self-reflection, calm thoughts, and establish connections between emotional systems and regions in the brain that are responsible for language. The authors write, "When the arts become a regular practice—the way you might improve nutrition, increase exercise,

---

[6] Bessel van der Kolk, MD, *The Body Keeps the Score: Brain, Mind, and Body in the Healing of Trauma* (Penguin Books, 2015), 244.

and prioritize sleep—you unleash an innate tool that helps you navigate the peaks and valleys of your inner life."[7]

Artmaking can be used specifically to address the aftereffects of trauma. One study of soldiers returning from war revealed that when they experienced flashbacks, the Broca's area—one of the brain regions responsible for language—literally shut down. Their brains resembled those of stroke patients, whose lesions in the Broca's area rendered them speechless. However, individuals with damage in this part of the frontal lobe are still able to make visual art—which becomes a tool to bypass the limitations of language. When these same soldiers participated in an art-therapy program to express what they went through, they were able to begin talking about what happened, and their PTSD symptoms lessened.[8]

There's also evidence that regularly engaging in the arts benefits people with physical pain. Illustrating what's happening in their bodies stimulates the release of healing chemicals, offers the potential for greater social support, and more. It even reduces the risk of developing chronic pain as we age.

By now, the scientific evidence is clear—the arts rewire our brains in positive ways. Besides benefiting patients and clients, all of these double-blind studies and qualitative analyses may finally influence policy makers, insurance companies, and medical institutions to include the arts in clinical settings. While the mammoth structure of society slowly develops and approves treatments, people who struggle from the effects of trauma have to find relief in real time. And while society is still playing catch-up, it's clear to those of us who have tried it that artmaking helps a great deal.

---

[7] Susan Magsamen and Ivy Ross, *Your Brain on Art: How the Arts Transform Us* (Random House Publishing Group, 2023, Kindle edition), Location 513–518.

[8] Magsamen and Ross, *Your Brain on Art*, Location 1303–1337.

WHY CREATIVITY?

There are so many other benefits to creative practices that can't be mapped through scientific measuring. What about that mysterious energy—that magic that keeps us coming back again and again to worship on its altar? For artists, it's the beckoning Muse. For those who self-harm, it's the promise of relief. Are they really that different? Is there a way to tease out the creative part of self-harming from the act itself so we still get that charge of relief without damaging our bodies?

As Mary Oliver wrote in her *Poetry Handbook,* "Poetry is a life-cherishing force. And it requires a vision—a faith, to use an old-fashioned term. Yes, indeed. For poems are not words, after all, but fires for the cold ropes let down to the lost, something as necessary as bread in the pockets of the hungry."[9]

Rather than turning to creativity as a simple *replacement* for our self-harming behaviors, perhaps we can see it as a method of digging deeper—a continuation, an expansion, a fulfillment of the work our deepest self is calling us to embrace. It can harness that divine energy in a way that is safer not only for our bodies, but also for our souls. Part of us knows that this secret ritual we've been repeating is not the right way in. It's limited. It keeps us stuck in a rut. It imprisons us in lonely cells where our sustenance is delivered in small doses, cutting us off from the source of nourishment itself.

And so, the answer to all of these questions is *yes*. The act of self-harming *is* creative and spiritual in its yearning, and we can mirror those impulses with healthier behaviors that will permanently rewire our brains. There are other ways to tap into the relief we get from self-harming, using creative methods. And the result will turn out to be a much bigger, more authentic connection to that energy of release, because it will be part of a bigger Energy, that spiritual

---

[9] Mary Oliver, *A Poetry Handbook: A Prose Guide to Understanding and Writing Poetry* (Harper Collins, 2024, Kindle Edition), 122.

force (or whatever you want to call it) at the heart of Creation itself. As a tremendous problem-solver and transmutation machine, it will change your self-harm into self-love. It will lead you back to yourself. And once you're there, nothing and no one can take that away again.

I know this because I've done it. And I'll tell you how I got here.

My Experience

Even though I was only four at the time, I can still recall today the sound the safety pin made as it scraped back and forth across the skin of my forearm. That's what haunts me, still—not the sight of blood, or the hot inflammation, but the *noise* echoing inside my body.

When I showed it to my mother, I claimed my little brother (not even two at the time) had scratched me. She didn't respond in any memorable way. That characterized much of her interaction with me in those early years—a sort of harassed impatience, as if I'd interrupted her private thoughts. She was consumed with her own unhappiness—unless she was consumed with her art, which was the only thing that seemed to make her happy. That incident with the "scratch" was my first conscious knowledge that I couldn't turn to her for help. Whatever message I'd tried to convey with that act had disappeared into a well of indifference. I was left to figure out on my own why I felt so uncomfortable inside *me*.

That first self-harming happened in front of a mirror. Apparently, I often stared at my reflection in those days. Mom used to tell me that whenever I cried, I ran to the mirror to watch myself. I spent long spells in the bathroom, dressing imaginary wounds on my skin. Whenever babysitters arrived, I'd emerge from the bathroom covered in bandages, moaning in pain. I'm not sure if the adults were amused or embarrassed, but I didn't get the effect I wanted—no one came to my rescue.

I felt unspoken pressure to avoid bothering either parent with my troubles. The rules were unpredictable, punishments unavoidable. So, I became more secretive with my self-injury. I banged my head against doors and stabbed my palms with pencils. My chaotic behaviors in school got me in trouble, an attention I hated but also needed. Inflicting my own wounds brought calm, even power—but also fear and shame. The urges felt so much bigger than me.

When I was nine, our house burned down. Soon after, we traveled to Europe for my father's sabbatical. It was in a castle in Bergen, Norway that I first heard a voice tempting me to jump to my death. It took all of my strength to resist. When we returned to Ohio, after I turned ten, my parents rented a place in town while our home in the country was being rebuilt. It wasn't just any place—it was a well-known haunted house. The stories of ghosts fused with the abuse, and my self-harming became more frightening. That year, when I was ten, I dug out my last baby tooth with a rusty nail. As blood ran down my chin, I searched the mirror for answers. I knew I should feel *something*, but a heavy anesthesia had entombed me, and there was no "self" in the eyes that stared back from my reflection. The horror of that scene was merely a distant echo as I hid deep in my psyche.

My little brother Andy had his own struggles. Even as a baby, he raged and cried with a strength that surpassed his tiny body. At two, he punched through a glass door, and at the hospital, five grown men had to hold him down so they could stitch the wound that ran from his wrist to his shoulder. A few years later, a dog bit a deep gash in his cheek. Adults labeled him "accident prone" because of all the things that mysteriously happened to him, leaving a trail of scars across his body.

Andy and I fought like devils throughout our childhood. We each became the stand-in for the parent we weren't allowed to hate. We lost ourselves in fistfights; we tore up whole rooms with our rage. Once we fought so hard that we got kicked off the school bus and had to find our own way home. In my young mind, he and I were equals—but I was his older sister, and later in life, he shared with me how much it hurt that I treated him so badly.

He also shared what he went through at the hands of our dad—at least what he could remember, which wasn't much. Over the years, we compared notes about the long beatings, elaborate punishments for imagined wrongs, fueled by accusations that seemed designed to pit us against each other. Andy always insisted he wasn't hurt the same way I was—until he heard me give a public talk in our old hometown about how I'd used my art to heal from sexual abuse. That night, the memories came pouring back to him, and he admitted it had happened to him too. But he had nowhere to put it in the tangle of addictions that were taking over his life. He died just six years later of complications from a drug overdose. He was only 52.

I didn't remember the sexual abuse until I was twenty-four. As soon as I got sober from drugs and alcohol, it all flooded in. That's what it feels like when the doors in your mind open up after being closed for years—like a great wall of water rushing through the corridors of consciousness. It finally made sense why I'd started self-harming at age four and wanted to die by the time I was nine. I remembered the sadistic punishments and humiliations, the killing of animals, the gaslighting (*Why are you making me hurt you?*)—but those were drops of dew on a web, not the actual spider.

At twelve, I had no conscious memory of the sexual violations that had happened to me from ages four to ten. All I knew was that by the time I was twelve, something had shifted. My dad, who was otherwise loving when he wasn't abusive, was disappearing into his alcoholism. My mom was disappearing into her stress about his alcoholism. I was edging into puberty. My one pal, a professor's child like me, was gone for her father's sabbatical semester—and so that year, I had no friends. The other kids teased me. I didn't fit in anywhere. The pain grew unbearable.

Then I read *I Never Promised You a Rose Garden* by Joanne Greenberg. The main character slashed her arm with a sharp object to vent the pain, and that sounded appealing to me. I took a razor blade from my dad's shaver and dug it deep into my young forehead. Once again, I did it in front of the mirror. Like I had with the baby tooth, I stared at the blood pouring down, wondering why I didn't feel any pain. But this time, I felt powerful, proud, and most of all, I felt relief.

That was the beginning of the formalized ritual that stayed the same throughout my cutting years. Whenever the urge came over me, I closed the door, faced myself in the mirror, and spent five to ten minutes dragging a razor deeper into my skin—first on my forehead, then my inner arms. I used the same blade, the same rag to gather the blood. I kept band-aids ready to dress the wound when I was done. I stored all my "instruments" in the same place in my closet. In my later teens, after a suicide attempt, I used self-injury to keep from killing myself—resulting in the largest scars along my inner forearm. In my twenties, I expanded to my wrists and ankles. Later, when I relapsed in my mid-forties, I cut the seams of my fingers.

Aside from doing it in front of the mirror, another commonality was the after-care routine. That became a time to nurture myself, to clean and cover the wound, then treat it gently until it healed. That was when I felt the pain—which filled me with warmth toward myself. It was a way to access a natural sense of nurturing that I hadn't gotten from my parents.

So, the very act of self-harming was creative. It was a way to communicate something that couldn't safely be expressed in words, an SOS code to summon rescue. It vented anger that I didn't know how else to handle. I learned from someone else's example and adjusted it to suit myself, then I created a ritual around it. Looking in the mirror became a way to search for answers to questions that didn't have words. I learned to take care of myself *through the act of self-harming*.

I also connected the act to music. I'd started playing violin at age nine, and the concertos, sonatas, and symphonies evoked deep feelings that I didn't know how to process. In high school, I fell in love with the music of my time. I got my first record player (long before CDs or streaming), and I begged, borrowed, or stole to get the albums I needed. I found that certain songs triggered a trance-like state, and I began playing those during self-harming sessions. That repertoire grew over the years, as I got older and started making my own money. Later, when I began conscious efforts to stop cutting, I played those songs while painting to redirect that internal energy. It was like coaxing the asp with seductive music so I could charm it into doing my will.

I was fortunate that my parents fostered an atmosphere of creativity. My father was a set and lighting designer for the theater, with a secret passion for architecture. My mother was an artist. Her mediums ranged from painting to quilting and fabric arts, and she let me use her colored pencils whenever I wanted. She also indulged my forays into candle-making, *papier maché*, flip books, and playing any instrument I chose. Both parents loathed television, so we rarely had one that worked—which forced us to create our own games. Andy and I built elaborate forts out of the snow and defended our kingdoms with snowballs. We fashioned wonky treehouses and transformed shipping boxes into spaceships. When the weather was bad, we draped sheets over the living room furniture to make a warren of tunnels. He took apart all the electronics in the house and built robots out of cardboard boxes. I constructed haunted houses at Halloween and carnivals during the summer, where I charged a nickel to play midway games.

Mom bought me my first Dungeons and Dragons set when I was twelve, and into that soup of depression shone a beacon of light. I was already bullied at school for being a nerd, so I kept the game secret and corralled my brother and his friends to play with me on the weekends. I became obsessed with the world of fantasy. When I was nine and then eleven, on two different sabbaticals, my father took all of us to Europe, where we lived on a shoestring and explored old castles and cathedrals. It was there that my sense of the world opened up beyond our little Ohio town. D & D brought that into my interior. I designed and illustrated my own campaigns, complete with original monsters, unique environments, and characters that became part of me. Their torments were more real to me than the confusing realities of teenage life. Simply drawing scales on dragons dropped me into a meditative state for hours and lifted me out of the misery that gripped most of my days.

My rich imagination, fed by my parents and the environments we visited, gave me a way to understand what was happening inside. I named that mysterious being that took over me "the Cutter." It felt male, supernatural, and huge. While I watched from far away, feeling no pain, that being did the work of self-harming.

I didn't yet understand what would later be termed "dissociation." My young nervous system couldn't handle the abuse and all the confusing messages that came with it—so it split into fragments to survive. One of those parts embodied the abuse—it carried the memories, the experience, and the reaction all in one. The cutting was its way of communicating. It would take me another four decades to finally stop, turn around, and ask what it was trying to say.

I used the same creativity that created that part to find my way back in to rescue it. I've often heard people say (in some form), "You can't use your brain to fix your brain"—well, that's not true. It just took a different part of my brain, the creative side, to find openings in the walls I'd built to protect my psyche. Whenever I drew dragons and knights fighting, I was trying to depict the battles going on within me. Later, when I started to paint, I documented my feelings through expressionist imagery. That act also defused the pressure that would otherwise lead to self-injury. Those artworks taught me things—they gave voice to the Cutter, to the experiences I'd left behind. Long before I shared my work with therapists, I was using creativity to process internal states, to find solutions to overwhelming problems.

Which brings us to the first of many paradoxes in this process—*the wound holds the answer*. The Cutter is also the healer. The solution lies within the problem. Those who abuse us the worst teach us the greatest lessons. And the journey to find and heal the broken part of us creates the skills, the gifts, that the world needs from us.

The gifts my parents gave me were exactly what I needed to heal from the wounds they inflicted, even though it took me years to appreciate them because the damage was so deep. I nearly succumbed several times, but I emerged with lessons to offer those who are still struggling. I wouldn't say I'm completely "healed"— what I am is stronger in the broken spots, better at asking for help, and more able to share what I've learned. By helping others, I keep the loving energy of healing moving through me and out.

Andy lost his battle too soon. But he left behind two beautiful daughters who carry his strength forward. Even though I couldn't save him, maybe with this work, I can help others in his honor.

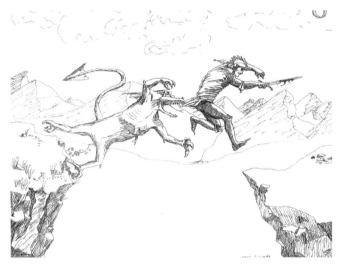

Figure 1: One of the many drawings depicting battles and chase scenes from my teenage years. Ink on paper, 1983.

Your Experience

By now, you may be wondering how all this could apply to you. My journey was specific to me and my experiences, in a specific culture and time. But how can *you* use creativity to help heal your wounds?

It starts with getting a sketchbook or journal—one that you'll use just for the exercises in this book. There are several reasons for that. First, it mirrors the ritualistic aspect of self-injury by creating a new sacred space for this inner work. Second, some later exercises in this book will utilize the work you did in previous ones, so it's more convenient to have it all in one place. It will also be useful to see the progression over time. And finally, it's just cool to have a book of your recovery—a testament to the work you'll be doing within these pages.

Not everything will fit in the journal. Some activities call for bigger pieces of paper, or other materials. You could always photograph those works and print out images to insert into your book. Or you could fold bigger pages into smaller shapes. Either way, try to store everything together. You may not believe me (yet) when I tell you that our artistic creations hold energy, but trust me, they do—and you'll want to honor and contain it.

Now let's address the subject of creativity in your own life. Perhaps you already identify as an artist of some kind and feel comfortable with the tools of a particular medium. Or maybe you don't think of yourself as creative at all, and the idea of being coached by a professional artist seems intimidating.

In my experience, I have found that artistic skill is roughly twenty percent talent and eighty percent training. We can all learn to draw, paint, sculpt, write, sing, dance, or act out a part. Some are better than others at any given activity, but it's part of human nature to communicate through language. And art *is* language. We've been illustrating our experiences for as long as we've been around, on any surface we can find, from cave walls to canvases and clay.

At one point, we chose self-harming as our go-to creative tool. By slowly re-directing ourselves into other mediums, we can more effectively (and safely) share our pain in a way that connects with others and heals ourselves.

Most of the exercises in this book are geared toward the visual arts. That's what I know how to teach. However, *any* medium that taps into your creativity will help in this process. Knitting, embroidering, dancing, singing, putting on a play—anything that connects your hands and eyes to the stories brewing inside, and gives you a new way to voice them.

Having said that, let's try an experiment.

Often, when I tell someone I'm an artist, they say, "I can't even draw stick figures."

Well, that's just silly. Everyone can draw stick figures. I dare you to draw one now. Just a ball, a line down from that, then two branches for legs, and two for arms. Stick figure—done. Now, here's a trick. Draw another circle, and this time, draw two lines down from that "head." Connect them at the bottom, and now you have a torso. Draw tubes instead of lines to flesh out arms and legs. Put little ovals at the end of each tube and now that figure has feet to stand on, hands to grab with. *Voilà*, a real person.

Here's the best part: in that circle head, put two dots for eyes, and a slit for a mouth. Next to that, draw a few more head circles and change the mouth and eye shapes to create different expressions—sad, surprised, angry, excited, confused. Add eyebrows to enhance the feelings.

Now, doesn't that communicate all you need right there?

To take it even further, draw two more head circles, and put eye dots and mouths in each one so they're looking at each other. Draw dialogue bubbles above each of their heads and write out a conversation they're having.

Voilà, a comic.

As it turns out, it doesn't take much to communicate through art, does it? In fact, I'm often the worst at games like Pictionary. It takes me ages to render something—while the non-artist next to me draws the clue in seconds, using rough marks. Sometimes, the simplest drawing is the most effective. We all have a natural ability to tell stories, and it's easier than we think to use visuals to communicate.

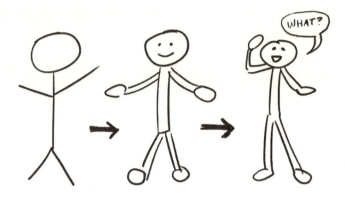

Figure 2: Anyone can draw a stick figure. From there, it's only a few more lines to create emotion and dialog. Give it a try!

Even if you're already an artist, I encourage you to do all of the simpler exercises so that your inner child can come out and play. So much of what we'll be doing involves communicating with our kid (or kids) inside, so we need to be able to let them emote without feeling judged for their skill level.

This isn't just a silly notion I came up with because I love doing art and want you to try it with me. There is so much evidence now about how our brains change when we engage with the arts. It increases our neuroplasticity, or the creation of new synaptic connections, and it also stimulates the brain to prune connections that no longer serve us. The stronger the saliency, or sticking power, the stronger the new connections. If we create the art ourselves, plugging into our emotions and utilizing our senses, we're amplifying the saliency of the re-wiring.

I'll leave it to scientists to map which cortex or network is being fired up when I create. All I know is that I feel power coursing through me as I "get it" through my visceral experience. I can sense my mind laying down new tracks. And that's the only thing that lets me know it's safe to let go of the old ruts.

WHY CREATIVITY?

There's one more aspect of this work that we should address now. In order to disarm our resistance to doing inner work, we need to tap into our own innocence—the part that is comfortable with spontaneous creativity. For so long, we've been taught by the field of psychology to think of it as our "subconscious"—as if we're ruled by mysterious internal forces outside of our control. But after doing the work I describe in this book, I've come to realize that there is no unconscious part of me—there are only parts I haven't yet accessed, parts that were shut away to survive a turbulent childhood.

There's a lot of shame in our culture about the whole inner child thing—it's often considered "woo woo" or regressive. And yet, weren't we all kids once? Did that inner kid just disappear once we reached our full height? And what happened to all their unresolved, unvoiced, unmet needs?

Befriending the child within may make us feel vulnerable to more abuse. But the difference between then and now is that your inner child is not alone anymore. They have you—the adult self, who, by now, is growing in maturity. We may think that past trauma has rendered that child forever broken, unable to heal old wounds. But those very traumas can be healed if we look at them with open eyes. The little one survived into adulthood after all, and they're eager to connect with us and others. Paradoxically, finding and embracing that innocent one is what gives us the strength we need to defend them.

If you still find it difficult to let go and connect with the littlest part of you, there may be another protective voice trying to keep that from happening. It learned to think critically and enforce others' rules to keep pain at bay. That voice is there to keep you safe. We'll address the subject more in later chapters, but for now, let's try a simple tactic to disarm it.

Picture some other kid you love—maybe your own child, niece, or nephew. Imagine how they'd respond if you told them they're being silly for drawing stick figures. Now extend that to your own inner child. Is that how you want to talk to them? We model our own critical voices from those who were mean to us growing up. Is that who we want to emulate? If we're criticizing and berating our little one inside, we're being abusive.

So, let's move forward with a spirit of openness. The exercises in this book will be much more productive if we let go of internal criticism. Curiosity is the mainstay of creativity.

Exercise: Listening Doodle

As with any new behaviors, it's best to start with fundamentals. If you've already drawn stick figures, you're on your way. Next, we're going to practice the art of listening to your drawing.

I learned this from my mother. She used to have art students put a mark on a blank piece of paper and ask that mark what to put down next. Once that was in place, she'd have them ask the next one what *it* needed. And again, over, and over. In that way, the lines would emerge from inner prompting. The skill of fashioning an image into a finished piece would come later; the listening came first.

I do my own version of this whenever I doodle. I like geometric shapes—drawing them soothes me—so I prefer journals with gridded paper to keep my lines straight. I start with a line or shape, then I let it decide what shape it wants next. Then I draw more shapes and lines until I feel finished. Sometimes I fill the whole page with a cacophony of geometry. It keeps my creative mind entertained when I'm in a meeting or watching TV. It soothes my nerves.

My mom also helped me develop my responsive skills in other ways. When we lived in the country surrounded by cow pastures, two miles outside of a college town with less than a thousand residents, she didn't have anyone to give her feedback about her art. She'd often call me into her studio to offer suggestions. I didn't know what composition looked better than the others, or what fabric would best complete a quilt, but when I simply asked clarifying questions, she chose the best direction herself. All I had to do was hold the space and listen.

So, try this yourself. Start with any piece of paper. It doesn't even need to be blank—it could be a magazine page or an office memo. Draw a shape you like. Don't judge, don't control it. Just let your hand wander and draw what it wants.

Now look at it, and pose the question gently in your mind, *What next?* Accept the first thing that comes and draw that. Maybe it's connected to your first shape, maybe it isn't. It might be a response to what's already on the page, if you've chosen a piece of paper that isn't blank. Just start drawing and listening and drawing and listening. Lose yourself in the doodle until you feel done.

You might also try this same exercise using language instead of lines. Start with a word, write it on the page, then ask it what word comes next. But don't just write it—create a shape with that word, one that interacts in some interesting way with the first one. Maybe it's looming over it or dripping down, one letter at a time. Or perhaps it's way off in the upper corner, turning away in fear. Let each word call out the next one; draw them into a visual poem. Let what comes out tell you what poem it's trying to make.

This technique could be carried into other art forms, such as dance. It's a skill I wish I had (but don't, sadly). However, that hasn't stopped me from dancing to music in the privacy of my own room, letting each movement dictate what comes next. The body is a powerful tool of expression.

Creating involves listening. We're not just blurting out any line and letting it stand unedited. It's an exercise in interactivity. It's how we become present with the work and with ourselves. We fuse new connections in the brain by making connections with what we're creating. We let the voice begin to say what it wants.

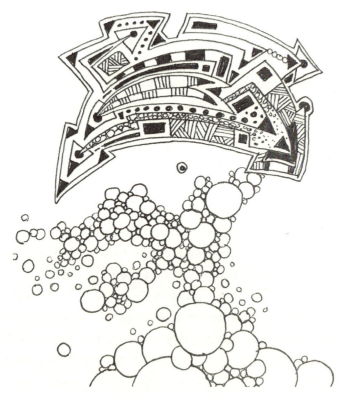

Figure 3: One of my "Listening Doodles," where I drew one circle, then another and another, then switched to angular lines, until it felt complete.

Exercise: Emotional Coloring

If you're intimidated by color and how it works, there's no need to be afraid. This isn't a course on color theory, and you won't be quizzed. It's just an exercise to find out which colors resonate with you and why. In the process, you'll get comfortable working with them in a more personal way.

We're going to adapt an exercise used by minimalist painters in the 1950s, except we're infusing it with that agent of saliency—emotion.

For this, you'll need a variety of color pencils and gridded paper. If your journal pages aren't lined or gridded, use a ruler to draw horizontal and vertical lines until you have a field of squares.

Choose any color you want and use it to fill in a square. Now look at that square and ask how it makes you *feel*. Angry, annoyed, bored? Happy, soothed?

Pick another color that evokes a similar emotion. Fill the square next to it. Fill in a few more adjacent squares with those first two colors, in no particular order. Try adding other colors on top of those squares. See how each addition changes the image and the feeling.

Now look for colors that are different from that first theme. If you initially chose red, you might head toward green or blue. Fill in some squares in a different part of the page, away from your original focus. Experiment with creating new combinations.

After you feel done with that area, start connecting it to the squares you started with. What colors best connect them? Is it a subtle gradation, or a jumble of all the colors you haven't tried yet? Does it cause anxiety? Is it fun?

Traditional color theory, and countless scientific studies, maintain that reds are associated with heat, passion, even upset and conflict. But not so in China, where red symbolizes abundance, celebration, and pride. In many cultures, black is associated with death and funerals; but in India, white has those connotations. Blue might feel soothing to many, as it's lower in frequency when it comes to light waves and can evoke images of water. It was also the rarest and most expensive hue on an artist's palette until synthetic paints were invented. And yet, if you were abused in your bedroom as a child, and your bedroom walls were blue, it's not going to feel comforting at all.

A few years ago, I had lens replacement surgery on both eyes. I opted to do one at a time, rather than both at once. After the first procedure on my left eye, the first thing I noticed was that the new lens perceived color perfectly, while the old lens in my right eye had yellowed. I had no idea I'd been looking at the world through an amber tinge. And yet, if you'd challenged my perception of color then, I would have defended my view as being right while yours was wrong.

That experience taught me that each person's relationship with color is unique and personal. It's influenced by our physiology, yes, but also our memories, culture, and preference.

What is your favorite color? And why does it make you happy? What colors repel you? Do they remind you of something negative from the past? Be open to learning new things about your relationship to color.

Exercise: Writing with Pictures

During my second trip to Europe when I was eleven, we went to see the Bayeux Tapestry in Normandy, France. It's a 230-foot-long embroidered story of the Norman Conquest of England in 1066, displayed lengthwise in one piece. Stitched into the cloth were sword-wielding knights, battle scenes, royals and ladies, boats, horses, and castles, accompanied by Latin narration. It was like an ancient comic, and I loved it. It stuck with me more than anything else we saw in museums, because it was telling a story. That's something I wanted to do.

I never became obsessed with comics, but I have created a few over the years, and I find it to be the best way to tell stories. They're like little movies. And they don't need to be complicated to be effective or therapeutic.

Now that you've drawn heads with dialog bubbles, creating a full comic is just a short step beyond. The easiest way to start is to draw out a series of panels. Each will be a separate scene. I find that six on one page is a good start.

Think about a simple story you'd like to describe. Maybe something benign like what you did when you woke up this morning. How would you draw a person waking up in bed? With a head circle resting on a horizontal line? Keep it simple. Above your head, write the thoughts that you had upon waking. You could draw a thought bubble around the words or leave them alone.

Now you have Scene One.

What happened next? Did your pet jump on your chest? Were you late? Did you have to rush out without eating? Illustrate that in the next few panels, along with what you said or thought.

Try to conclude this little "story" with a final scene that sums up how your morning went. Put that in the last panel. This way, you have a narrative with beginning, middle and end on a single page.

It doesn't need to look professional or make sense to anyone but you. My friend Diana is a writer, not an illustrator, and yet she creates the most amazing comics depicting ordinary events. The important thing is that by telling a visual story, we're infusing it with structure and meaning—and perhaps seeing something that we didn't notice before.

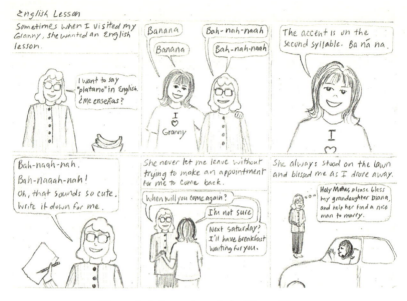

Figure 4: A 6-panel comic by Diana Flores, who doesn't consider herself an "artist," but who exemplifies that innate creativity we all carry.

Advanced Exercise: Try On New Outfits

If you already draw or paint on a regular basis, it might seem silly to draw stick figures and color your emotions. But I encourage you to do these exercises anyway. See if you can tap into your childlike joy as you do them. Make a game of it. How simple can you make your figures and still convey the human form? What *are* your favorite colors, and why? How does each make you feel? If you hate a particular hue, why is that?

Do you doodle? And if so, which patterns emerge most often? Can you introduce something new? Try doodling whenever you watch television or sit in a meeting—just mindless scribbling with minimal conscious effort. Engage with the drawing only to ask what comes next. Let go of the reins.

Take a cue from the minimalist painters and create a geometric composition using only colored shapes. One of my teachers in college, Karl Benjamin, had his students cover a canvas with a grid of squares in different hues. It was comforting—the only decision I had to make was which color fit next to the one I'd just painted. If you're an intellectual creator, this activity can help you bypass the thinking brain and tap into the feeling part.

You could try "comic journaling" for a month. Pick an event that happened to you from each day and illustrate it in six panels. Do it as simply as possible. After you've done a few of these, you'll start to notice themes in how you see the world, what grabs your focus, how you tell stories.

Another way to approach this is to do an exercise popularized by the artist Roy Lichtenstein, who copied comic panels in oversized paintings. Select a single panel of your own comic and develop it into a much larger piece, using your favorite medium. See if you can get to the emotional essence of that panel. Let the sheer size of the image turn up the volume. How does it feel to blow open that moment, to step inside and experience it in a new way? Is it frightening? Does it make you laugh?

The goal is to tap into that automatic creator inside you—the child's viewpoint, unfiltered by outside messaging. Artists from Modernism onward have been searching for ways to unlearn their artistic training and get back to the spontaneity of childhood creativity. Paul Klee called it, in his *Pedagogical Sketchbook*, taking the "line on a walk."[10]

---

[10] Paul Klee, *Paul Klee: Pedagogical Sketchbook*, Trans. Sybil Noholy-Nagy (Frederick A. Praeger, 1953), 16.

Suspend judgment and find your own way in. Anything that builds trust in your Muse will aid in this process of healing.

Reflection

Every time we finish a stage, we're going to reflect on it. This is as important as the exercises themselves. Self-harming is a method of containing chaos—so as we re-train our neural pathways, we're going to have to pause along the way and organize our thoughts. Writing about feelings connects the brain's two hemispheres—the right side, which processes emotions and abstract thought, and the left side, which is responsible for language and writing.

So, write about your insights thus far. What is it like to view your self-harming as a creative act? What happens to your energy when you change your viewpoint from shame and fear to curiosity and willingness?

Is the self-injury a response to trauma from your childhood? If so, what might the wounds be trying to say?

Practice letting your pen express whatever it wants. Doodle or color any time you feel like it. Draw a few stick figures and let them dance around, talk to each other, and amuse you with their antics. Decorate your notebook with patterns. Let the line take you on a walk.

Another important part of the process is to share it—with your therapist, counselor, or guide. They might be able to see things you hadn't noticed. Also, communicating with someone else solidifies learning pathways. As the saying goes, if you want to learn something, practice it; if you want mastery, teach it. By teaching others about who we are inside, we make it more real. Our true self begins to emerge from the shadows of our secrets into the light of our unique, creative selves.

Concluding Thoughts

In this chapter, I made a case for creativity as a therapeutic modality. We learned we can harness the creative aspects of self-injury to re-train our responses and build new neural pathways toward reaching for art instead of self-harming. By starting with some basic exercises to flex creative muscles, we're easing into the process. There's no need for any purpose yet, other than the joy of making marks on paper. This is a new way of doing things, so be gentle and go slow.

In fact, that's a good mantra to keep in mind from now on—*be gentle, go slow*. Often, going slowly is, counterintuitively, the fastest way to get somewhere. We're used to the chaos of uncontrolled energy, overwhelming emotions, and category five storms. It takes time to unwind those tornadoes. Let these simple exercises draw out that thread, one turn at a time.

In the next chapter, we'll prepare for the journey. Does that sound ominous to you? Corny? Are you curious, excited, nervous, skeptical? All of the above?

If you're feeling more nervous than excited, remind yourself that this is just a book. If you want to, you can roll your eyes and throw it in the trash. Alternatively, if you're open to it, you can use it as a guide to help you forge a new path away from self-harm into healing. Deep inside, part of you wants this. Otherwise, you wouldn't have read this far.

Doubt, fear, and impatience are all to be expected. Faith is required to walk this path—faith in yourself, in your future, in the possibilities that lie beyond what you know.

It takes time to do this work, and lots of help. Let's move on together, but remember, *be gentle, go slow*.

"When I use my strength in the service of my vision, it matters less and less whether I am afraid."

—Audre Lorde

"There are no signposts in the sea."

—Vita Sackville-West

CHAPTER THREE

PREPARE FOR THE JOURNEY

Since we're being gentle and slow, let's first pause and gather what we'll need for this work. Every time we go on a trip, we pack. We think about what we'll need, we plan for what could go wrong. Maybe we buy travel insurance or a new swimsuit. We check to make sure our license or passport is up to date. If we have a specific routine at home, we research how to carry that with us—if our gym has a branch in our destination, if our 12-step group has meetings there. We read about the adventures that await us, plan side trips, find new restaurants. Even those of us who hate planning still put gas in the car and throw clothes in a suitcase.

I've learned over the years that no matter how well I plan (I'm a big fan of lists), I always forget *something*. All I can hope is that I'll be able to replace that missing item at my destination—or that I won't need it after all. Recently, when I went to visit my mother in her remote town in Upper Michigan, the airline lost my luggage—for *three days*. I decided to just go with it. I wore her pajamas and shopped for outfits at the local Walmart. When I finally got my suitcase back, I felt like a new person.

Anecdotes aside, this upcoming journey *is* like losing your luggage on the way to revisiting your childhood. It can feel uncomfortable and unfamiliar. No amount of planning will fully prepare you for the experience.

But there are some essentials you'll need before embarking.

The first thing to do is enlist help. You'll need someone who can act as both witness and advisor. I've made my case for working with a therapist—preferably a professional who has experience with self-harming behaviors and training in mind-body work like Somatic Experiencing or EMDR. But not everyone has (or wants) that kind of resource. The important thing is to have someone nearby who cares about you, and who won't judge or pressure you to stop if they get scared. They have to be safe enough that when you feel triggered to self-harm, or feel ashamed if you do, you can reach out to them for help.

The second is to think about what could go wrong. What is your "insurance?" If you veer too far into the bad neighborhood inside your head, what can you do to come back? What will you do if you slip? If you get overwhelmed, what is your escape route? Take some time to think about that and write out ideas.

My best escape is sleep. When I get overstimulated, I take a nap. I work at home, so it's not much of a stretch—but even when I worked at a company, I utilized their private lounge next to the women's bathroom when I needed to shut down for twenty minutes. There have been times when I found myself too upset to drive, so I pulled over and napped in my car until I could safely continue.

Exercise helps as well, although I don't always have the energy or motivation. Sometimes the phone, which has the power to connect me to others, can weigh a thousand pounds. So, putting on a familiar meditation brings me back into myself—especially guided meditation through ear buds. Several popular apps offer free visualizations. I choose the ones with the most soothing voices or nature sounds.

Somewhere along the way, I also discovered that listening to binaural beats helps to regulate my moods. I used to download tracks from different online sources. Now, it's easier to find free recordings on apps like Insight Timer. The binaural beats come in various frequencies, which are calibrated to enhance different activity levels, from creativity to sleep. It's another form of bilateral brain stimulation that mirrors EMDR or Butterfly Tapping.

When I first started this work, I had no control over how deep I'd go or for how long. My therapist taught me somatic techniques and mindfulness exercises to ground myself whenever I felt triggered. I played with different breathing techniques to calm my chemistry. The simplest, and my favorite, is the one that I learned from my dog. Phoebe can nap anywhere, anytime. When something disturbs her rest, she heaves a big sigh—and slips right back into sleep. So, I do that too. I inhale all the fear and emotion and hurl it all out in one exhale. I call it the *dog sigh*. It works every time.

Phoebe, and my cat Shilo before her, taught me that simply surrendering to the process relieves a lot of the stress around it. So much of my anxiety was caused by resistant thoughts: *Why is this happening? Will I ever be free of this? How can I make this go away?* Once I accepted, without judgment, that I'd be in crisis for however long it lasted, it became easier to do whatever was in front of me. I committed to doing the work on a regular schedule, five days a week. Having a consistent time, with a clear beginning and ending, smoothed out the ups and downs of my internal world, because it reassured all my internal parts that were clamoring for my attention. Once they knew that they'd get the attention they needed, it became easier to focus on the daily tasks of adult living.

That evolved into a daily habit of morning check-ins. What I do with that time has changed over the years; but it always connects me with my deepest self. Whether I'm employing meditation, prayer, visualization, writing, artmaking, or all of the above, I'm communicating with the Spirit inside and outside of me.

When I say "Spirit," I'm referring to my own personal version of what many call God. Sometimes I use that word too. Some prefer to use more neutral terms like The Universe, or Nature, or higher power. If you're reading this book, you're probably open to the idea of a spiritual energy that can be accessed through creativity. If you're not, the upcoming exercises will help you find what works best for you.

Just remember, there's no rush. *The fastest way is to go slow.*

My Experience

In my own path of recovery, I had to find signposts in a sea of confusion. Before there were books, or online resources, or therapeutic modalities about cutting, I turned to art. I drew for hours. I read poetry and attempted to write some of my own. I listened to whatever soul-moving music I could find. I devoured books, television, and movies—anything about moving from darkness into light.

When I was a teenager, fantasy novels, especially by Tolkien, fueled my imagination and inspired illustrations. *Moby Dick* and *Heart of Darkness* made me realize that other people are haunted by despair, too. History books opened my eyes to the wider world of humanity. Alice Walker, Toni Morrison, Zora Neale Hurston, and many more taught me about dignity in the face of injustice.

But it was Ursula K. LeGuin's *Wizard of Earthsea* that resonated most deeply during those years. Its protagonist, Ged, is a headstrong young student at a wizard school (long before Harry Potter). During a competition with a hated classmate, Ged's prideful showing off accidentally summons a demon into the world that nearly kills him. He tries everything he can to escape it—until he finally gets sick of running and decides to confront the demon, even if he dies in the process. A loyal friend helps him pursue the wraith beyond the edge of maps into the open sea. There, he finally grabs it, turns it around, and diffuses its power by saying its true name, "Ged." With that, he embraces the demon and enfolds it back into himself. I've seen that archetypal path mirrored in other stories, including the *Star Wars* series and *Six Feet Under*—but LeGuin's novel is still my favorite.

This concept of an internal demon reminded me of the Cutter. That being took over me, controlled my body, and numbed my pain. When I read LeGuin's book, it was still the early '80s, and no one (least of all me) used words like "dissociation" or "depersonalization." There was only what I experienced, which was a sense of being unreal. I never knew when I'd be sucked out of my world and into an alternate place, where everything looked and sounded scary. I couldn't even trust reality.

Drugs and alcohol helped. Once I discovered that when I took a handful of the Tylenol + Codeine I'd been prescribed for bronchitis, the emotional pain disappeared. I didn't just take one or two—I took as many as I could without throwing up. When I couldn't find regular drugs, I took bottles of aspirin. It was less about getting high and more about self-poisoning. Same with alcohol. I didn't want to drink and end up like my father, who'd become the notorious town drunk—so when I did take up the bottle, it was to degrade myself. Fun came eventually, when my friends caught up, and I became the cool one who could snag "supplies" from my father's pockets. I was able to crawl out of my isolated hole into a semblance of popularity, but the specter of despair haunted me.

Self-harming, self-poisoning, and a growing addiction to substances weren't enough, so I added bulimia to my dysfunctional toolbox. Promiscuity came naturally, since I'd never been taught to say, "no," and my drinking put me in unsafe situations. More often, the line between consent and refusal blurred, and my shame only deepened.

And yet throughout high school, I maintained straight As. I became captain of the swim team, concertmistress of the county orchestra, head of the yearbook committee. I won competitions and praise. No matter how much I achieved, though, nothing made me feel worthy of love. The sensation of unreality lurked on the sidelines, ready to take over at any time.

One afternoon, as I stood in our kitchen, *Every Breath You Take* by the Police came on the radio, and I felt a heavy presence inside me, watching me, just like in the lyrics. I knew in my heart that it would never leave. Discouraged, I leaned against the wall—and I couldn't move. Time disappeared. I stood pinned to that spot for what felt like hours, terrified at the helplessness in my own body.

A suicide attempt at seventeen alerted adults that I was in crisis—and finally, a teacher stepped forward to help. Mrs. Hren was the first person who gave me hope. She and her husband went above and beyond to take care of me. Once during a snowstorm, they picked me up at the end of my long driveway and took me to their house to watch funny movies. She told me that one day, I would be grateful that I didn't succeed in killing myself—and she was right. With her love and attention, I was able to avoid a hospital stay, get back to my studies, and eventually land a full scholarship to a college outside Los Angeles. I remained close with her for the rest of her life.

Knowing I was going to California gave me the courage to acknowledge that I might be gay. It started with a "might" because I was afraid. Friends had already warned me that if anyone they knew turned out to be gay, they'd be ostracized. But I wanted to find out for myself. I went to softball games. I got a fake ID and visited the gay bar an hour away. I knew in my heart this was the real me, but it would take another seven years to stop sleeping with men.

When I got to college, I discovered that my despair came with me. It reached a new level of anxiety. I sought help from the school clinic, but I couldn't connect with my counselor, so I ramped up my other coping mechanisms to get through college and into a job. Once I had medical insurance, I was able to find a therapist, who worked with me on and off for the next twenty-three years.

Soon after starting with her, my drinking and using spiraled out of control. The morning after my worst binge, I called a sober friend who took me to a recovery meeting. I slowly let go of my addictions—first alcohol and drugs, then bulimia, and eventually, self-harming. With the help of my creative practices, I maintained that cease-fire for many years.

But when my twenty-year relationship began to fall apart, the self-harming returned with a vengeance. By then, my therapist was nearing retirement, and I sensed that I needed a different kind of help. She'd been trained in traditional psychoanalysis, which is steeped in dogma and maintains strict walls between clinician and client. The mental health field had gone through a sea of change toward humanistic practices, informed by discoveries about the effects of trauma.

They say the teacher will come when the student is ready—and this time, I found the therapist who would lead me safely into the place beyond maps where I could finally meet my Cutter—and heal the long-frozen wounds inside.

Through all this, I gained valuable lessons. Suffering from trauma pushed me to search for relief, which gave me experience in building my own toolbox, however dysfunctional at first. The isolation of my childhood led me to books, where I received guidance from other peoples' stories. Because I was so lost, I learned to ask for help. Desperate to stop self-harming, I imitated the rituals in my painting and channeled that energy into productive new behaviors.

Which brings me to the second paradox of spiritual healing—*the trauma creates the tools we need to heal from it.*

This is why you don't need to have any special talents to harness creativity in your healing. The tools are already in your arsenal—they were created by the need to heal in the first place. They are unique to you. And they belong to you alone. All you need is to consciously assemble them into one place for easy access. Pack for the trip.

And don't worry, whatever you forget, or whatever you don't have already, will appear when you need it. You're more resourceful than you could ever imagine.

Your Experience

There are five main steps in this process of preparation:

1. Assemble a TEAM.
2. Create a place of SAFETY.
3. Gather the TOOLS.
4. Create a new RITUAL.
5. Affirm your IDENTITY.

TEAM

Although we are the only ones who can do the inner work to get better, we can't do it alone. Thankfully, the field of psychology offers many modalities and resources, and a simple online search can lead us to the right practitioner, program, book, or workshop to help us heal from trauma. As I've said, I'm a firm believer in therapy. I couldn't have done the deeper work without a skilled therapist. But I also have other people in my life who care about my well-being. I had to enlist all of them as I trudged through recovery. Looking back, I realized I was never alone. I had a team of people cheering me on.

You'll need one too. To assemble your team, list out your resources. Who have you asked to help you along the way? Who is your main guide today? Who are your safe people? Write out their names and contact info. For me, that list includes my therapist, recovery sponsors, and partner. I used to have a psychiatrist on that list. As a teenager, I only had my counselor and Mrs. Hren—but they were invaluable, and they kept me alive. Writing out their names reminded me I wasn't alone when I was going through the worst of it. So, identify your team and stick close to them. Make sure they know where you are on your journey.

SAFETY

Next, we need to create our safe place—inside as well as outside. Since I love naps, that place is usually my bed. Sometimes I can get that comfort just by covering myself with a blanket. When I'm out in the world and can't just go to sleep, I hold onto a talisman of some kind—usually my sobriety coin or my favorite necklace. The important thing is that I have a physical reminder of the haven *inside* of me.

I have many visualizations and practices that help me experience safety within my body, regardless of what's happening in the world around me.

An early one came from my therapist. When she first expressed verbal affection toward me, I told her it felt overwhelming, so she had me imagine myself inside a plexiglass box where the lock was on the inside, and only I had the key. I could see and hear her, but I could keep her outside the box until I was ready to let her in. Instead of just visualizing the scene, I went *inside* my body to experience the physical sensation of being safe.

She taught me visceral techniques like this, informed by her training in Somatic Experiencing (SE). Created by Peter Levine, Somatic Experiencing is a powerful mind-body modality that addresses the problem of trapped chemistry—that physiological trauma residue that can't be accessed through talk therapy alone. He observed that many animals become immobile when faced with danger—then when it passes, they tremble violently before resuming their active state. He surmised that people who had gone through trauma experienced a similar paralysis and needed to have a subsequent release to return to normal.

Levine stated:

> Any animal that is trapped in a situation where fight and flight are not viable options will use [immobility as their first line of defense]. Another of the vital functions of the immobility response is numbness. If the impala (or human) is killed while "frozen," it will not suffer pain or even terror during its demise. We humans use the immobility response—frozen energy—regularly when we are injured or even when we feel overwhelmed. Unlike the impala, though, we tend to have trouble returning to normal after being in this state. The very feelings that

we need to access in order to...help steer ourselves back to the present are, in effect, numbed-out.[11]

Levine developed different techniques to help people "unfreeze" their trapped energy, process physicalized emotions, and return to calmer states. My therapist shared them to help me ground myself in my body. By focusing on an internal experience, and describing its location, texture, shape, and other qualities, I was able to connect that physical sensation with an embodied *me*. I was able to loosen the energy that had gotten "frozen" along the way. Sometimes, big chunks would release and burst through me at once—usually during therapy, but sometimes at night—so I had to learn how to regulate that flow. My therapist guided me safely through the rapids until I could steer the boat myself.

Whether or not we were abused as children, self-harming also creates trauma in the body—and as we embark on a journey to heal from it, we need help with releasing the chemistry. Most therapists who are trained in trauma-healing modalities will use mind-body techniques like SE or Eye Movement Desensitization and Reprocessing (EMDR) with clients. Meditation apps like Insight Timer or Calm offer guided visualizations to aid in grounding.

When I was still self-harming, my therapist and I came up with agreements about what I'd do during surges. When I felt a strong urge to self-harm, I agreed to let her know. Usually, I'd make a commitment to abstain that day. By that time, I trusted the boundaries of our relationship enough to keep that commitment—and I never broke it, not even once.

This is a good time for you to create some guidelines with your therapist or guide—agreements about what happens if you

---

[11] Peter A. Levine, PhD, *Healing Trauma: A Pioneering Program for Restoring the Wisdom of Your Body*, (Sounds True, 2008, Kindle Edition), 34-35.

self-harm during this process. What that entails is up to you. The important thing is that *you* feel safe. Our interiors may be chaotic, and we don't want to jump right into them without emergency contacts at the ready.

TOOLS

Third, we gather our tools. Not the old tools, but new ones, just for this upcoming work.

Many of us who have self-harmed have, at one point or another, kept a favorite blade or sharp instrument. Some might keep it in a special box. When I used a blade to cut myself, it was then considered "active." An active blade had far more power than a neutral one, and it had to be kept wrapped up. I often stored it in a special place alongside band-aids and rags.

Do you have a particular tool that you use in your self-harming?

To do this work, we're going to need *new* tools—creative ones, starting with the journal I recommended earlier. If you haven't already, assign a special pen to use in that journal. Those of us who infuse our self-harming tools with imagined power need to assign our new tools equal importance. You might want to decorate that special pen, or wrap it in a band-aid, or otherwise mark it as a tool to be used by the hand that does the self-harming. Since we're going to be using color, it might be helpful to purchase a set of colored pencils reserved for these exercises. Each time that pen or pencil executes a creative act in this book, it's adding to the power inherent in that tool.

RITUAL

This is sacred work. Creative acts connect us to the greater Creative Intelligence of the universe in a tactile way. Not only do we need special tools for the fourth step of preparation, but we also need a new ritual.

What do you do to prepare to self-harm? Do you put on specific music? Do you lay out a particular towel, wear certain jewelry? Does it happen in front of a mirror? It is important to acknowledge our rituals, because as we build new ones, we're re-training our minds and bodies to forge pathways to healing—using the very routes we rode to self-harm. It doesn't work to just replace the behavior with something else. If that worked, I would have been "cured" when one of my early therapists suggested I pound a pillow instead.

So, this time, honor your process instead of hating yourself for it. Buy a new towel or piece of fabric to lay out under your drawings. Get that special pen or set of pencils. Buy a candle to burn while creating. Wear an item of clothing just for this work. Sit in the same chair each time. Make a new music mix, more upbeat and hopeful.

Set up a schedule for doing inner work and stick to it. Maybe ten minutes after coffee every morning. Or Sundays from 4–5. When I finally committed to working with my inner parts, to getting to know myself once and for all, I scheduled one hour a night, just before bed. That was when my anxiety was highest and my chemistry most activated. I would read material on what I was going through, then write or draw. On the nights when I didn't feel up to it, I still spent the time with myself, soothing my inner parts. The rest of the day could be spent on work, family, errands, personal stuff, recovery activities, whatever—but that daily hour was sacred. If I had to skip a session, I acknowledged to my interior that it was just a schedule change, and I'd be back the next day, as promised.

If it's too chaotic inside to commit to a regular time, then just agree to do the creative work whenever you feel like self-harming. Or whenever there's an upset in your chemistry. Create a system that works for you.

IDENTITY

Remember the last thing we do when packing for a trip? We check that we have our license or passport—that identity marker that is recognized by the outside world. Before embarking on this inner exploration, we need to reaffirm who we are today, as adults.

Make a list of who and what you are in the world today. Use every label and description you can think of—be truthful, but kind. For example: I am an artist, designer, author, teacher, and mentor. I'm married with two fur babies. I'm queer, in my late fifties, American, of half-Finnish and half-British Isles descent. I'm sober and active in my recovery. I'm an incest survivor who used to self-harm, and I use what I've learned from my healing to help others. I've been a swimmer for over forty years. Recently, I've become an Airstream camper, something I never envisioned.

Sometimes, I list my favorite things in different categories—movies, books, colors, places I've visited. It helps ground me in a self that exists here in the world, today. Plus, as I've said, I'm a big fan of lists. Feel free to create your own library of favorites.

This prep work is the first step in organizing our lives and our interior worlds. The act of self-harming is an attempt at controlling chaos—now, we're going to learn new ways to do that. By redirecting that raw energy, we'll train it, mold it, and enlist it to serve us as we move forward.

So, let's begin.

Exercise: First Steps Inside

During that special time that you've set aside, with or without music, open your journal. Hold your special pen. Close your eyes and breathe gently through your nose, into your belly. Feel the energy in your body—in the skin, nerve endings, arteries, muscles, bone. Touch on the breath moving into your lungs, then travel through the organs. Now sense yourself inside—the presence that is you. Feel its shape, its edges, its substance. Let it be what it is, without judgment of control.

Follow it through your body. Gently summon it into the pen in your hand.

When you're ready, open your eyes. Using that pen, and the energy contained in it, draw the "you" that you tracked inside. Don't think, just draw. Let whatever shape comes out just be what it is. There is no perfection here, no need for likeness. Draw until you feel done, then close your eyes. Breathe. Now open your eyes and look at the image. Greet it with gratitude.

If it doesn't look like anything, or you don't like what you see, thank it anyway. Thank yourself for being willing to do this. No matter what comes forth from inside us, it's worthy of our love.

Now, write a few words to describe how you felt inside. Describe the drawing itself. This time, instead of thinking about who you are to the outside world, you're paying attention to who you are inside. Does that sense of self feel hollow, haunted, fluid, solid, sparkly, dissipated? What color is it? What temperature?

We may present a certain persona to the world, but if it's detached from our interior, we'll always feel "off." I used to tell people I felt like a Warhol print—off-register, misaligned. I couldn't connect my inner personhood with the outer me. It wasn't just distracting—it was crazy-making.

This and other exercises in this book are intended to help us reconnect with ourselves—and see which bridges need repair.

Exercise: Mapping the Journey

You might want to use a bigger piece of paper for this one. Use the special pen and/or colored pencils.

Draw yourself about three quarters across the page—the "you" of today. You may have an outer representation with a different image inside it, or you might just be a stick figure.

Now, go to the left side of the page, more toward the upper half so there's room beneath it. Moving from left to right, list or draw the markers of your life thus far—where you were born, houses you lived in, school graduations, relationships, breakups, jobs, and whatever life events shaped the "you" that bears your name. Create physical landmarks to represent those events—maybe a school building for your graduation, or a hill you climbed to achieve something. Try to end at the present day around three quarters of the way across the page, leaving some empty space on the right. Draw a line through those events and connect it to you. This is your outer journey thus far.

Return to the starting point at the left side of the page. In the empty space below that, start to map out your inner journey, moving from left to right. Maybe it begins before birth, with the events that happened while your mom was pregnant. List or draw your internal atmosphere as your childhood developed. Mark the realizations, big feelings, betrayals, discoveries, joys, and sorrows. Get creative with how you represent the more abstract states—maybe a swamp where you slogged through a depression, or a cyclone that swept you into chaos, or an explosion that tore you apart, or a sun that warmed your face for a time. Continue all the way to the present, connecting the line to the "you" of today.

Take some time to study the two trajectories. Where are they connected, where are they disjointed? Where did an event on one line influence the other? What are the differences and similarities between the two maps? You might want to draw lines connecting some of them.

Under each of the milestones, both outer and inner, write the lessons you received from that experience. There will be obvious ones, like professional skills you received from getting a degree; then there will be more subtle ones, like learning patience when you didn't get a job you wanted. Draw an icon next to each one that represents that tool.

Now we're going to map out the future. Starting with the present point, which is (hopefully) about three quarters of the way through the page, continue each line toward the right edge. You can probably sense what the road looks like in the immediate future, because it will most likely be a continuation of what you experience now. But since it hasn't happened yet, we're free to imagine whatever we want.

Where do you want the inner journey (that lower line) to go? What changes would you like to see? Draw the things you hope for, letting go of doubt and fear. This is a drawing, not a declaration etched in stone. If you weren't afraid, if things went your way, if there *is* light that you can't see yet, how would your path change? Conclude it with a drawing of your internal self that has achieved all that you could hope for. Connect the line from the current inner "you" to the future one. Imagine encountering an obstacle (like the critical voice, *That'll never happen*), and draw a tool or weapon that might combat that foe.

What about your outer path, the one on the top half of the page? How will it be influenced by the inner journey you envisioned? Allow yourself to dream big. If your inner self has grown and changed, discovered new hope, overcome fears, and found healing, what might that bring into your outer life? Would you find work that you love, maybe a healthy relationship? Children? A new career? Or are your goals more abstract, like "success" or "helping others"? Can you see the new tools that will result from the inner work you've done? See if you can connect the two lines along the way so the internal and external goals are one.

When you get to the future Inner Self, draw an Outer Self around it. Use words and/or imagery to describe that person. What would that unified Inner/Outer Self say to the "you" of today?

Advanced Exercise: Call On the Muse

My writing teacher, Adele Slaughter, teaches her students to take the Muse seriously. She has them write the Muse a letter at the beginning of each session. It has to be dramatic and flattering, like, "O Muse, beautiful one, grant me the gifts of your bountiful creativity."

It felt silly the first time I did it, but somehow, it worked. My work flowed easily.

After a few years of writing those Muse letters, I had an intense dream about a powerful transgender being who went around pushing into peoples' foreheads to open the third eye. They created little children and fantastic constructions of magical materials. They put one of the children inside a wooden structure that looked like a religious triptych—where it died. I cried over that terrible loss. The transgender being came over to me and opened my third eye—I can still remember that sensation on my forehead—and said, very clearly, *My name is Obedon.* And suddenly, I understood that the child (creation) had to die out so something new could be born in its place.

Okay, so my Muse is a transgender destroyer who opens my consciousness. (Someone once teased me, "Why must your dreams be so cryptic?") After that vision, it made sense why I always illustrated surreal beings from my subconscious. I was trying to capture this mysterious energy that drives me to create. I don't question it anymore. Now I simply call upon Obedon to guide my thoughts, hands, and eyes every day, and I have a continuous source of energy for my art and writing.

Who is your Muse? If you're resistant to the idea, can you approach it with an open mind and heart? Just try it. Sit down and write a letter to it, starting with the salutation, "O Muse." Say a little prayer inviting your creative source to come visit.

You can try illustrating it. If you have a particular type of music that induces an otherworldly mood, play that while you work. Use the automatic drawing technique you tried in the last chapter and let the image flow out through your pen or brush. Is your Muse male, female, other? Human or animal? Are there tools, weapons, decorations, symbols? Give yourself over to the process, and don't judge the outcome. If nothing happens right away, wait, and try it later.

Another way to access it is to find images that appeal to you and collage them into a portrait. It will be made up of the things/people/inspirations you love. Who is that being? Is it a guru, trickster, mother, guide? Can you frame it and hang it near your workspace, then call upon it every time you create?

If you've taken the time to ask and are patiently listening, the answer will come, I promise.

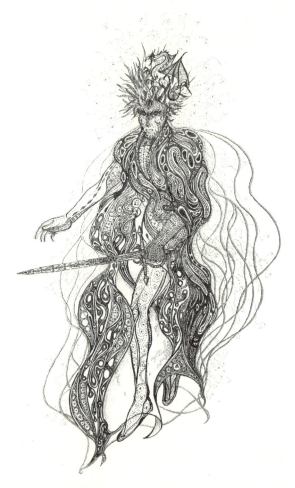

Figure 5: "Mr. Blue," an early drawing I did of what turned out to resemble my Muse. Ink on paper, 1987.

Reflection

After you've done the exercises, write about what you learned. Track the lessons. Share it with someone.

Describe what it feels like when you acknowledge, assemble, and hone your tools to fashion the life you want. Do you sense more power inside? Can you describe that feeling beneath your skin? Are you more confident in this process or still skeptical, hopeless, or fearful?

Answer this question: What would you be doing in your life if you were no longer afraid?

How is your self-care? Do you have ways to ground yourself in your body, people to call when you need help? What areas need work? Take some time to make the lists suggested in this chapter. Make verbal or written commitments to yourself and someone else. You don't need to rush anything. Just do what you need to take care of yourself and take it slow.

Is there a creative being or source of energy that inspires you? If you don't have one yet, can you sense it coming?

If something stood out, simplify that into an affirmation or mantra. For example, if you saw that you have indeed made good choices along the way, say to yourself, "I know how to make good choices," or "I trust my inner instinct more and more." Look to your own experience for the tools you already have. Honor your strengths. Enhance them. You're writing the handbook of your own life.

Concluding Thoughts

In this chapter, we focused on five things that need to be strengthened before we dig deeper—team, safety, tools, ritual, and identity. By evaluating yourself, how you got here, and where you're going, you're containing what feels chaotic. Grounding techniques, both somatic and creative, will keep you steady in the recovery process. Instead of looking at your self-harming and the traumas that it caused in a negative light, you can begin to see how you've developed positive traits as a result of it. This builds resilience and inspires hope.

We also discovered that *the trauma creates the tools we need to heal from it.* The skills you need are already present inside you—because if you're self-harming, you're trying to heal yourself, and you've developed strengths as a result. Those particular tools are well-suited for a creative sojourn.

Remember to be patient and go slowly. My hope is that by sharing my tools with you, your recovery time will be shortened—but it takes what it takes, and there's no rush.

The antidote to fear is faith, but those of us who've struggled with feeling unreal often struggle to have faith in anything. It takes real courage to trust in a hopeful future you can't yet see.

If it's harder than ever, that's a good sign. It often gets harder before relief comes. Just keep going. The gifts will far outweigh the pain—in fact, they will give the pain meaning.

You aren't alone. There is someone there, holding your hand, waiting for you to squeeze their hand back. It's time for you to meet them.

"Perhaps everything terrible is in its deepest being something helpless that wants help from us."

—Rainer Maria Rilke

"From the ideal to the archetype! Presumptuous is the artist who does not follow this road through to the end. But chosen are those artists who to this day penetrate the region of that secret place where primeval power nurtures all evolution. There, where the central organ of all temporal and spatial mobility—call it brain or heart of creation—activates every function; who is the artist who would not dwell there? In the womb of nature, at the source of creation, where the secret key to all lies guarded."

—Paul Klee, from the Jena Lecture, 1924

CHAPTER FOUR

THE CHILD AND THE SPIRIT GUIDE

A lot of research has been done regarding how children attach to caregivers and the world around them, the effects of trauma, and the particulars of the developing brain. Some studies have been shockingly cruel—like Harry and Margaret Harlow's experiments with rhesus monkeys in the late 1950s. They showed that when babies were separated from their mothers during the first year, especially after being subjected to stress, they engaged in self-mutilating behaviors like biting and slapping themselves, banging their heads, or trying to chew off a limb. Other experiments proved that young monkeys need to attach to caregivers, even if they're just wire structures covered with cloth. When their mothers were subjected to emotional and sexual torment, these parents ignored or even killed their offspring.[12]

These psychologists were able to demonstrate (and label) concepts like "learned helplessness," "insecure attachment," and "generational trauma." But no one seemed to notice the elephant-sized

---

[12] Marilee Strong, *A Bright Red Scream: Self-Mutilation and the Language of Pain* (Penguin Books, 1998), 48-50.

question sitting in the middle of their labs: *Do we really need to torment animals to prove that mistreatment leads to problems in childhood development?*

Rather than experiment on animals, some researchers have paired them with people to see if they could heal each other. Programs like equine therapy for troubled youth, horse training in prisons, and pets in hospital settings have generated reams of proof that working with animals reduces symptoms of PTSD and aids in healing.

It seems the hardest concept for researchers to embrace has been simply asking people what happened to them. Freud was not the first or last doctor to turn away from his patients' truth and use the architecture of science to re-frame it to please others. The psychologist and philosopher Alice Miller argued that Freud acknowledged the effects of trauma when he wrote *The Aetioleogy of Hysteria* about his female patients' sexual abuse at the hands of their male caregivers. But after being ridiculed by his peers, he pivoted and formed the Oedipal theory, which placed the onus of blame back on the child—the adults didn't abuse them, those were just fantasies the children created to deal with their confusing sexual attraction to (and competition with) their parents.[13]

And yet, once again, no one questioned the elephant on the psychiatrist's couch: Why was Oedipus at fault for marrying his mother and killing his father?

The answer is that he wasn't to blame. He didn't know those people were his parents. No one told *him* who he really was.

---

[13] Alice Miller, *Thou Shalt Not Be Aware: Society's Betrayal of the Child*, Translated by Hildegarde, and Hunter Hannum (The Noonday Press, 1998), 41, 322.

My Experience

When I was struggling with unnamable feelings, with no access to the buried memories, the field of psychology was just barely—and reluctantly—beginning to deal with the concept of post-traumatic stress. It was sort of accepted that soldiers in war experienced it, but it took many more years to acknowledge that children did, too. The same year I started cutting myself with razor blades (1979), Alice Miller published her groundbreaking *The Drama of the Gifted Child*, one of the first professional-authored books to vouch for abused children. Progress in the '80s and '90s was slow and steady, as more psychologists and psychiatrists focused on patients' childhoods, rather than relying solely on diagnoses and medications. Federal courts began to re-shape laws to honor victims of child abuse, remove statutes of limitations, and award damages. Books about cutting appeared on the shelves—some by clinicians who'd helped clients heal, some by people who'd recovered.

Bessel van der Kolk's book *The Body Keeps the Score* wasn't published until 2015, bringing the word *trauma* into public discourse. It's still a best-seller today. In 2021, Oprah co-authored *What Happened to You?* with Bruce D. Perry, carrying the subject further into popular culture. These and other authors describe how hard it's been to overcome resistance in the field of mental health, as well as in public opinion. The temptation to dismiss the child's experiences runs deep—which makes sense, given how many people use denial, aggression, and blame to cope with their own experiences.

Along the way, backlash was often brutal. Sensational stories and erroneous accusations of Satanic abuse fed media tropes about the unreliability of childhood memories. In 1992, Dylan Farrow accused her father Woody Allen of sexually abusing her and was ridiculed in the media. Most people, in public at least, blamed her accusations on the vengefulness of her hysterical mother. Even those who had sympathy for her qualified it with the understanding that children often exaggerate, or they misremember things, or they're easily influenced by adults' hidden agendas.

But I believed Dylan. Even before I read the in-depth articles about the case, I knew she was telling the truth. I could see it in her body language. When she gave interviews later, as an adult, I recognized her struggle to verbalize, to avoid being flooded, her regret at having to upset others while remaining firm about what happened. I'd experienced all of that and more.

About a year after remembering the abuse, I wrote my father a letter confronting him with what he'd done to me. We didn't talk for the next seven years. During that time, he sent my brother a fifty-page letter (actually, twenty pages with thirty more of footnotes) declaring his innocence in all things parent-related. He blamed my hysterical mother for influencing me with her victim story. He said he'd joined the False Memory Syndrome Foundation, and after researching all the studies, he knew I must have been hypnotized by my therapist. He detailed every event of our childhoods with explanations about how he'd been misunderstood, maligned, and under-appreciated, referencing stacks of affidavits that supported his claims.

My mother didn't believe me, either. My accusations pitted her feminist beliefs against her fear of being blamed. She'd spent much of her adult life advocating for social justice—civil rights, women's rights, poor people, environmental issues—but was unable to see the victimization happening in her own house. The shame of that was too much to bear, so she just didn't talk about it. Andy followed her example and avoided the whole subject. So did everyone else in our extended family. No one *said* that they thought I was crazy—but by carefully avoiding any mention of my father or by avoiding me completely, each person conveyed their skepticism.

At the time, I felt angry at being dismissed by those who should have listened. It compounded my pain over not being protected when I was little. I couldn't yet see that they were part of the same culture of denial that had allowed the abuse to happen in the first place. I processed the feelings the only way I knew how—through writing and creating art.

My father maintained his innocence until the very end of his life, when he made a confusing deathbed confession that left more questions than answers. In one last burst of energy during hospice, he told his companion Frank that he needed to ask for forgiveness. Frank recounted it to me the next day, after Dad had slipped into a coma and could no longer talk.

Frank asked, "You molested Maggie, didn't you?"

According to Frank, Dad replied, "I didn't molest both my children."

Frank then asked, "Did you burn down your house?"

Dad replied, "Yes, I walked away from a burning cigarette."

Dad died two weeks later, and I was left to wonder what he'd meant, if he'd really said those things, and if he'd fully admitted to himself what he'd done before surfing into the great beyond.

Whether or not he intentionally burned down the house, he *did* molest both his children. Once Andy remembered the abuse and started talking about it, my mother finally began to believe me. I still felt upset with her for not acknowledging me earlier, but she just couldn't access it. She described it as a closed-off compartment in her brain. My brother's addictions kept her confused, worried, and hooked into his roller-coaster dramas. His final overdose left her feeling bereft and guilty. She sought help from others to get through it. In the process, she started facing what her husband did under her watch—and she courageously talked about it with others in her support group.

Andy's death in 2022 helped me achieve more compassion for my parents. Watching him progress from innocent kid into suffering addict gave me a glimpse of how cycles perpetuate in families if they're not stopped soon enough. I was able to see how the difficulties in my mother's childhood set the stage for her denial later—just as my father's early abuse twisted him into an abuser. I often say I'm in a "state of forgiveness"—which means I've granted compassion, but I can still get angry at times. I don't excuse anyone's actions. But I appreciate that my parents did the best they could. And I know how hard it can be to go against the grain of your upbringing and choose a new path.

In my experience, true forgiveness isn't something we engineer out of virtue or preference—it's a gift and often comes when we least expect it. But we can't jump to it without processing anger first. If the one who's been hurt is an innocent child, that child needs to be defended, rescued, and given a voice. If that child lives inside us, the only one who can do that is our adult self. Once we've put in that work, we might find acceptance, compassion, or even forgiveness—but as an organic aspect of spiritual growth. If it's forced in order to avoid feeling anger, it's rarely genuine.

As I stated earlier, not everyone who self-harms was physically or sexually abused. But somewhere along the way, the child inside was traumatized—by bullying, confusing messages, boundary violations, or neglect. That vulnerable being had to find some way to vent unbearable feelings in the absence of words. Language is what we use to communicate and connect with others. When we can't do it verbally, we find another way.

And so, any journey toward healing self-harm involves meeting the child within. Not just meeting them, but engaging with them, earning their trust, and listening to what they're trying to say.

This requires courage and a willingness to let go of resistance. Because let's face it, that denial that pervades our culture also lives in our brains. If the very thought of doing inner child work conjures embarrassment, that's a sign that you're on the right track—because that embarrassment serves as a sentry to keep you from going deeper. We're taught to "grow up" and leave the past behind, to stop obsessing about ourselves and "being a victim"—yet all those voices do is stop you from going further. They don't bring anything positive into your life.

Once you start the work, though, those warning thoughts will ease. The further you go, the more you'll want to continue. And you'll see that this is where you were always supposed to be.

Going Inward

I wasn't looking for a deep inner experience—I was just trying to stay asleep.

The nightmares had mostly subsided, but I was still sometimes heaved awake in the middle of the night. I was in a relative lull in my late thirties, I was solidly clean and sober, the Cutter was locked away, my relationship was humming along, and we owned a house. There were friends, parties, family gatherings, and occasional trips. I still fretted over my erratic income during that middle of the night. That, and the possibility of the house slipping off its foundation, or the brick face peeling off. Sometimes, I had to grip the bed so it wouldn't buck me out of it.

I'd stopped working on my recovery from drinking (I thought I was cured), and I only went to therapy for annual "tune-ups." Yoga and meditation were my primary means of personal reflection. I had to find something to get me through those three a.m. panic zones without waking up my partner.

So, I came up with a visualization.

One night, I envisioned a bedroom with a big cabinet that opened into an elevator, like a gateway to Narnia. I stepped into it and descended, counting ten, nine, eight, all the way down to one. The door slid open, and I saw a flat, open field with a forest beyond.

Even stepping out of the elevator was too much at first. My mind would skitter back into worries. Once I'd lost the image, I'd have to start again, counting down from ten until I returned to the field. Sometimes I fell asleep. Sometimes I gave up and just squirmed in anxiety until the sun came up.

After a few nights, I envisioned taking off my socks and shoes and leaving them in the elevator. For some reason, that freed me to step out. The wet grass cleansed my skin—then soft, lined boots appeared on my feet. I didn't seem to be in pajamas, so I clothed myself in a medieval tunic with leggings and a belt. I worried about that metallic elevator door disturbing the natural environment, so I had vines reach out and cover it. Then I worried about being able to find it again, so I had it light up whenever I approached. As each obstacle arose in my mind, I came up with a way around it.

The forest seemed scary at first, so for a long time I just rolled in the meadow, staring at the sky. If I'd made it that far without thoughts intruding, I usually fell asleep. Eventually, though, I was able to reach the woods.

It wasn't frightening, after all. It was calm and quiet and smelled of pine. I recognized that scent from the woods around my childhood home.

I noticed that I was much smaller. I could feel the compactness of my limbs. There were no scars on my arms. I was a kid again when I thought the whole world was magic. The forest was alive with spirit, aware of my presence. The trees dipped their branches to greet me.

One in particular called persistently—a wide, tall oak with gnarled roots. When I stepped closer, a door in its trunk opened to let me in. Once I was inside, the bark closed behind me, and I was safe.

I spent many nights furnishing that space, filling it with baby animals and soft pillows. I envisioned them in such detail that I could hear the kitten purring as it fell asleep on my neck.

When I was ready, I ventured out of the tree and deeper into the forest. Fairies pestered me as I walked. One of them landed on my finger. In the privacy of my mind, I didn't have to be embarrassed that my visualization contained fairies. I was traveling through the woods of my childhood into the Middle Earth of my imagination. I could feel the bark under my palm and hear the wind in the leaves.

I stopped in front of a cave entrance. The fairies took off in a fuss, so, of course, I wanted to see what was in there. I was that brave kid once again, exploring the ruined mines by our grandparents' house in Butte, Montana. Darkness and death didn't scare me. I entered the cave.

As my eyes adjusted, I could sense the bulk of a creature. It was a dragon, lying on a mound of treasure. It lifted its wings and uncoiled. The glow from inside its chest glinted off jewels and gold coins. But it wasn't evil. The Smaug of my early drawings, my knights' eternal foe, was now my guardian. He let me climb up and sleep against his stomach.

I got to be angry there. The dragon gave me a special sword and a mannequin to slash. It was self-healing, so every time I cut the head off, it snapped back into place. I could stab and slice to my heart's content. Sometimes, the dragon spewed flames until the mannequin shriveled into a lump of coal.

A lot of time was devoted to surveying my riches. When I was little, I'd bite the shells off M&Ms, divide them into color-coordinated piles, and eat them according to hue—so I did that with my imaginary jewels. I divided the garnets from the diamonds, the sapphires from the pearls, then mixed the piles so they all clinked together.

I'd read somewhere that you should never look into a dragon's eye, because that was how they gained power over you. But he told me I could ask him anything, and he'd answer through his eye. I could feel the truth of his words. So, I started asking him questions. He always answered with the truth. I, who couldn't even trust my own thoughts, could trust this fantasy dragon.

The last leg of the journey came after the cave. The path got darker; the trees loomed bigger. The sound of trickling water guided my way. There was a sense of presence, as if the forest was aware of me walking through it.

A clearing opened up ahead, just beyond a running creek. I stepped over rocks to reach the other side. My outfit transformed into a loose robe. My boots disappeared, and the water cleaned my bare feet. Ahead of me, sitting on a mossy bench, sat a radiant Being.

She was already familiar to me. I'd only ever seen her once, when I was seventeen, right after my suicide attempt. After I'd puked my guts out in the ER and the doctors had put me in a room to sleep, I drifted into a haze. Sometime in the night, the door opened. Light spilled into the room. I squinted and saw a nurse, wearing an old-fashioned white uniform and hat. But then she started to glow from within and she became more like an angel.

She spoke to me without moving her lips, "You're so beautiful. You don't need to do this to yourself."

A wave of peace filled me, and I knew I'd be okay. The next day, I realized it must have been a dream, yet it felt so real. Seven years later, on one of the worst nights of my drinking and using, I had a similar experience of a presence holding me. It helped me decide not to kill myself. Instead, I called the friend who took me to my first recovery meeting.

This and other experiences in sobriety led me to believe that the Being in my three a.m. visualization wasn't a dream character—she was my spiritual guide. Whatever that meant wasn't as important as the feeling itself. I knew it in my heart. I could recall the physical sensations and the great wave of peace. I began to call her Lady of Light.

She lived in that deepest part of the forest. I rarely got to see her, because I was doing this visualization to relax, and I usually fell asleep before I got that far. When I did reach that clearing, I'd go to her and rest my head on her lap or sit on the ground and lean against her knees. She stroked my hair. Any physical comfort I'd ever gotten, from people or animals, distilled into that visceral experience. It always delivered me into sleep.

It seemed the more time I spent rehearsing these internal wanderings, the more I believed they were real. I realized that each of these three stages corresponded with a different age. When I curled up in the tree, I felt the youngest. By the time I met the dragon, I was somewhere between five and ten years old. In the final portion with Lady of Light, I was a pre-teen or young teenager. As I imagined each scene, I was *in* it; yet over time, I noticed myself witnessing it, as well. That part of me noticed details, spun stories, and sifted out meaning.

That witness part was my conscious self. I began to call it "The Captain of the Ship." It's my everyday *me*—the one who's living my life, with all its memories and goals and adult problems. All three child parts report to the captain who steers this vessel. I can't do it alone—a captain relies on the crew to know what's happening throughout the ship. We all need each other to stay on course.

Without intending to, I'd spontaneously re-parented myself. No therapist told me how to do it or even said it was necessary. I simply wanted to find relief from pain. I followed my own promptings, through a pathway made up of my past experiences, guided by spirits that my inner child recognized.

When I finally found my new therapist in my forties, and shared that experience with her, she had many insights that helped explain my fragmented interior. She, too, had discovered on her own that we all have parts inside, and those who experience trauma often lose contact with them. Working with her solidified my belief in what I was experiencing. And I learned better ways to interact with my internal family.

This process of owning my inner child parts also led me to the "God of my understanding" that I'd heard about in recovery programs. It was no longer an abstract concept or a bearded guy in the sky. It was a real feeling inside my own body, one that I finally believed in—because it was embodied in the tree, the dragon, and Lady of Light. My little ones had led me to these aspects of Spirit. Even as they each relied on their own version, they knew it was part of a larger whole.

The lesson that came from this part is less of a paradox and more of a conundrum—in order to start healing, to rebuild broken trust, we have to ask the one who *doesn't* trust to have faith in something. That may feel like an impossible task. But if we don't go to that source of our internal disconnection, we'll never be able to heal.

The exercises in the next section are designed to take you to that source, to a place that is both childlike and spiritual. If those two energies have lost each other along the way, it's time for them to reunite.

Your Experience

I've guided many others on this path, and it always amazes me how simple it is. Once people are led into a visceral, personal experience of their inner world, they no longer feel silly about the idea of going there. That's because no matter how fragmented our psyches are, we can usually sense *someone* inside us—the child we used to be, the one who viewed the world with wonder. Before adults taught us about things like gravity, we believed we could fly. Before someone defined God for us and told us what we should believe in, we had a connection of our own. We came from a great soup of Spirit, the mystery that lies just beyond our conscious reach.

It felt a lot more real when we were still new to this world. That little kid inside *knows* what they do and don't trust. We can feel their acceptance or resistance in our bodies, in our gut responses. Even if we struggle with dissociation, there are moments—little strings of realness—that connect us to that source inside. The child will show us what to believe in.

Below are some exercises I've used to communicate with that child and to access their versions of Spirit. If you feel embarrassed or reluctant to do these exercises because of preconceived notions about inner child work, that's fine too. Use what you like and leave the rest. The important thing is to let your interior wandering take its own course. Just try one thing and see how it feels—and if it's okay to continue, try another. Once you make the connections, the path starts to form itself. Try to hold faith in that.

The purpose of these activities is to stimulate our own interior mirroring. In all my research about those who self-harm, there seems to be a commonality of not having adequate positive reflections from caregivers. We can find some measure of that later on with partners, but it's risky to rely on an intimate partner to hold the mirror for us—we give up some measure of personal responsibility in the process, and people are imperfect and will fail us. The only way to find permanent stability is to create a healthy mirror *inside you*.

Just a reminder: the reason for using creative exercises is to create new neural pathways. We're releasing old chemistry that's been encased in past trauma. Creativity and an open mind are the vehicles that carry us there. Suspending judgment is the most loving thing you can do during this process.

Grounding Technique: Butterfly Tapping

Developed as the "Butterfly Hug" by Lucina Artigas,[14] this tapping technique is a great way to self-soothe. It's one of the Bilateral Stimulation protocols used in EMDR. I use it whenever I'm heading into deep work that might be triggering or when I need to settle after being flooded.

First, hook your thumbs together against your sternum, with both palms resting just below the collarbones, one on each side. With your eyes closed, gently tap your fingers against your upper chest, alternating back and forth in whatever rhythm feels right.

---

[14] Lucina Artigas and Ignacio Jarero, "The Butterfly Hug Method for Bilateral Stimulation" (2014), https://emdrfoundation.org/toolkit/butterfly-hug.pdf.

Another therapist I know teaches this technique with a slight variation. Instead of fluttering the fingertips on the chest, she taps each hand twice—tap-tap, switch, tap-tap. Like a heartbeat.

Whichever rhythm you use, do it for 30-60 seconds, or until you feel a shift in your energy.

Visualization: The Child and the Spirit

The child needs to feel safe and heard, and the adult needs to let go of cynicism—so any visit between the two should start with a process to calm the body and mind. Think of it as a supervised visitation so that you can feel more comfortable meeting with them alone next time.

There are countless guided meditations out there for the child or children within. I encourage you to find what resonates most with you. When I work with people, I use the one I developed on my own. It feels most natural to me. You might want to read through it first, then follow the general directions until you find your own way. Or you can go to www.stoppingselfharm.com to listen to a free recording of this visualization.

First, set aside time where you won't be disturbed, and find a comfortable place to settle. It helps to cover yourself with a blanket. Treat yourself as you would a child you adore. If you're in bed, hold your pillow, curl up, get comfy. Breathe deeply and fully. Relax your face muscles. Agree to let go of resistance, but also, use your thoughts to follow a safe path. You're surrendering and staying in control at the same time.

I'm going to lead you on a similar pathway to mine, starting with the bedroom and the elevator. Imagine a safe place indoors. Decorate it however you like in your mind. Notice a mysterious door. Open it, and see an elevator car—an inviting space, gently lit, with your favorite song playing on speakers. Step inside.

The door slides shut and begins to descend. Watch the numbers light up—10, 9, 8, 7, 6, 5, 4, 3, 2, 1. Whenever your mind wanders (and it will), keep returning to where you left off.

Feel the elevator sink to the bottom floor. After a moment, the doors open.

Let the scene unfold. Maybe it's a field or a forest. Or maybe it's a beach. Maybe it's the moon! If it feels uncomfortable, exert your mind slightly to nudge the image toward a safe environment—someplace where you can feel peace. You're allowing and creating at the same time.

Once you have a scene that feels right, notice what you hear and what you smell. Let curiosity prod you out of the elevator and into this new world.

As you wander at your own pace, notice details of the landscape, what you're wearing, how your body feels, and so on. Let it be gentle and slow. Enjoy the newness of it. Let go of fear—nothing bad can happen here. You've entered the realm of your deepest self, that is untouched by the outside world. We all have it—trust it. Let it guide you.

Notice something calling you in a particular direction. It could be a sound, a glow, a yearning—or just something that's more charming than your thoughts. Allow yourself to drift toward it at your own pace. Observe your mind co-creating the scene as you go along.

You can see the thing that is calling you ahead. It starts as a blur, then as you get closer, it solidifies. It's familiar to you, just as the dragon was to me. Maybe it surprises you—maybe you knew about it all along. It knows you too. You feel a wave of unconditional love flow over you. See it more clearly now. Let yourself fold into it. Feel comfort on your forehead, around your shoulders. You're free here. Float in that space for as long as you like.

Either drift into sleep, or when you're ready, come out of it slowly. Either way, be gentle. Thank yourself for being willing to do this exercise. If you like, write down what you saw or draw it.

Or just hold it in the privacy of your mind. This belongs to you.

Keep returning to that place whenever you want. As you become more comfortable with the exercise, start filling in the details of your inner landscape. You are co-creating this story with your Spirit—the part of you that connects to the mystery, whatever that may be. There are forces at work beyond our comprehension. We create the avatar that represents that energy in a way that makes sense to us—whether it be God, Allah, Buddha, or Krishna, Nature, the magic of science, a dragon, a tree, Lady of Light, or an old man named Pluto (I've heard it all). The only thing that matters is that your inner kid believes in it and trusts it.

Exercise: Supervised Visits

Now that you have tentative contact between the little one inside and their concept of Spirit, take some time to draw them out (literally and figuratively). Get to know that little one, where they live, and what they feel. Work with them to enhance their contact with that source of spiritual comfort.

One of the classic ways to access the inner child is to engage it with non-dominant handwriting. But rather than jumping in with no context, set the stage first. With this and any subsequent exercises, put your journal and pen nearby, then take a moment to settle in, breathe, count down from ten, and enter your child's inner environment.

Once you have that visceral connection, open your eyes, and write out a question with your usual writing hand. Start simple with something like, "What do you like about that place?" Or "How are you feeling right now?" Then switch the pen to your non-dominant hand and write out the answer. You'll notice right away that you have to slow down and concentrate—like a child who is learning to spell. Try to quiet your brain's running commentary and let it flow.

Let whatever answer appears lead to your next question. For example, if you asked, "How are you feeling?" and the other hand answered "Worried," follow up with something like, "Why do you feel that way?" Don't try to fix it right away, like an anxious parent. Just listen.

Continue with the question/answer process until you feel done. Close it out by writing a warm thank you with your dominant hand.

Another method is to draw instead of writing. You'll start with the same process, but this time, ask the question out loud. Then draw (with either hand) the answer. Kids don't care if they demonstrate artistic talent—they create whatever they want. Let yourself be a child with a crayon again. Your verbal questioning voice is the compassionate witness. Start easy to set the child at ease. What do they like to eat? What's their favorite animal? What do they want for their birthday?

At some point, the questions may go deeper, and the answers might convey pain. Don't try to fix it or convince them everything is okay. Just be curious and loving.

When it feels like time to stop, let your adult draw something fun to make the kid smile. This shouldn't be hard—you know them better than anyone on earth. Thank them for being so honest.

Exercise: Engaging with Spirit

Before we begin, write some notes about your concept of Spirit. What is your current image? Do you believe in a godhead, or a universal intelligence, or a general sense of mystery? What did you visualize as a child?

If you could invent your own higher power, what would it look like? If you had no doubts or skepticism, no limits whatsoever, what avatar would you create? Write a list of the attributes it would have. Alternatively, if you already believe in God or Spirit, describe its amazing qualities. Set that list aside—we're going to return to it later.

Now, get into your comfort zone with the inner child and start to draw. Ask your kid to create an image of their Spirit. Feel it inside you—that sense of comfort and safety. Let it be a child's drawing of God—not one the adults superimposed, but the being they see when they feel truly connected. Try to let go of any religious constrictions. Draw truthfully and simply.

After that's done, ask the child to draw *where* they live inside your adult body. Let them render this configuration. Don't judge how they depict you—the important thing is to locate them inside the you of today.

Then have them draw the Spirit/God figure as it relates to the body. Is it a little squiggle inside the heart? Is it a membrane surrounding your aura? Is it a force in the sky shining down?

Make sure it rings true to the child.

When you have something that feels real, take a moment to feel the child where they dwell inside you. Greet them there. Sense the Spirit in and around you. Feel the child connecting with that energy. Track it through your adult body.

This is a physical connection you can draw upon at any time—while driving, in a meeting, watching TV. Once it's established, it doesn't require a prolonged ritual to drop back in. It belongs to you. It's as strong as you choose to make it with your belief and repetition.

Another way to make this more tactile is to sculpt a figure. If you have access to clay and know how to use it, that will work. For everyone else, I recommend purchasing some Sculpey modeling clay from an art store or online. It's a user-friendly material that can be baked to harden the form or left alone to dry on its own. It's easier than you think to sculpt. I once threw a Sculpey party, and everyone was amazed at what they could create without any "talent" or training.

Following the pathway outlined above, let your inner kid sculpt their version of Spirit. Whatever you create, the kid will enjoy the sensation of squishing and pulling the clay. It might be harder if you haven't envisioned a concrete being—in that case, think of a symbol or shape that would represent the feeling of Spirit, like a heart or star.

Or you could create a "pain rock." My mother went through a phase of researching and painting petroglyphs and connecting them with her ancestral Sami traditions. She discovered stories about sacred stones that were scarred from years of weathering. Some people believed that since those rocks had already been through so much, they were strong and wise enough to hold human suffering. So, they named them "pain rocks"—repositories for people to leave their troubles behind.

Feel free to form a simple lump and scar it with whatever instrument you choose. Once dry, Sculpey can be painted with acrylic. If you're feeling ambitious, follow the package instructions to bake the figure, then finish it with color. This is your process. If it's not too big, you can carry it around with you; or just put it in a special place so it stays safe.

I didn't sculpt my Spirit figures, I drew them—but I did carry around talismans. It helped to have something in my pocket or purse that I could touch whenever I felt uneasy. I still carry my sober coin with me, numbering the years since I've had a drink. It reminds me of what's real. Find something that brings you comfort—that reassures you when you're in upheaval, that communicates to your inner one that you're still there. Like a wedding ring seals our commitment to a partner, a talisman, chosen by the child and carried by you, signals that you believe them. You are their mirror.

Finally, take out that list you made of your higher power's attributes. Read it out loud, inserting the words "I am" in front of each attribute. *I am loving, I am kind, I am gentle.* Hearing yourself say these things reinforces *your* true nature. It offers a mirror to the inner child who didn't have a sense of self growing up. And it establishes what it *feels* like inside when you are aligned with Spirit.

Next time a critic inside your head says you can't do something, or calls you a name, ask yourself, *Is that word on my list of spiritual attributes?* If not, then it's going against what you know to be true at your deepest level. It's old programming, and there's no place for it anymore.

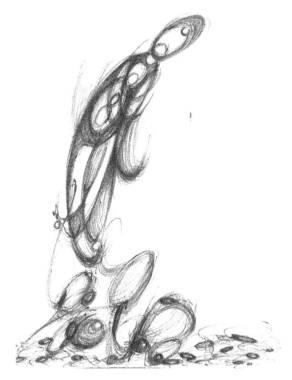

Figure 6: An early drawing of Spirit, done after a deep visualization.

Advanced Exercise—Self-Portrait with Spirit

You may have done self-portraits before, but this one is different. If you haven't, this will be a first—either way, it is an interesting way to explore your deeper self in the mirror. We'll be trying two different versions.

First, find a favorite photo of yourself as a little kid, at any age. Now, take a picture of yourself in that same pose as the kid from many years ago. On paper or canvas, sketch that outline of you today, leaving some empty space around it. Then sketch the little one inside, as a smaller version of that adult you. Where you place the kid is up to you.

Think about the child and the Spirit you contacted in the visualization. Using the references you chose, start to draw or paint your little one. Can you feel the energy of them inside? What's it like to see your own young face appearing in paint? Wait until it's materialized into recognition before you start on the adult you. How does this little one see you today? What is it like to sense your skin of today from within a much smaller form? How do the two connect—through lines, colors, images, or empty space?

When you're ready, shift your focus to the area around the figures. Imagine the spiritual being you met in the visualization. What would they be doing if they were standing right behind you, surrounding you with love? How would you indicate that in your rendering? Is it an encompassing angel, a bird on the shoulder, an aura, or a color? Let your hand go into autopilot.

Trust what comes out.

The second version of this exercise is more spontaneous. Set up your easel or drawing pad in front of a mirror so that you can easily see your reflection while you work. Take a moment to study yourself. How does it feel to look into your own eyes? Who's in there? Can you sense the little one inside, and if so, are they looking through your eyes too? If not, where are they?

Now, start to sketch yourself. Don't worry about getting a likeness. Hold in mind the child and the Spirit that you met in the visualization. Where are they inside your body, and how would they look in this self-portrait? Keep looking back into your eyes as you work. Connect to that energy. If it feels scary, or if you're not happy with what's appearing, ask for help from your Muse. Sketch their form around you. See if you can tap into a positive feeling like enjoyment, love, curiosity, or serenity. Work until you feel done.

After either of these exercises, study what you've created. You might want to wait a few days, then look at it again. Is there something in there you hadn't seen before? Is it pleasant, disturbing, inspiring, or confusing? Write about it.

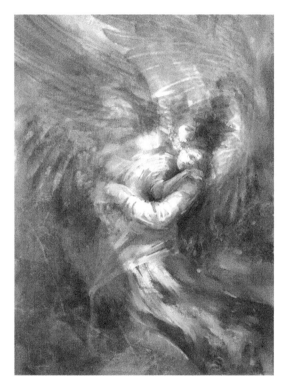

Figure 7: "The Father," 2012, depicting my spiritual version of the father I didn't have in real life. I started painting it in oil, then digitized it into Photoshop, where I added an old photo of Dad holding me. Then I printed it out and painted more on top.

Reflection

Once again, after you've done the exercises, journal about what you experienced—not just from your adult, analytical viewpoint, but from the kid's perspective. Give names to their impression of Spirit, of you, and of their interior world. Share it with someone who won't judge you. Show your child inside that you see them, you believe them. And you've got their back.

As with any relationship, it takes an investment of time and energy to build connections. Keep checking in. When emotions overwhelm you, check in to see what the child is feeling. When you feel wonder at the beauty of a sunset, ask the kid what they see. Treat yourself the way you would a beloved child of your own. Give them the gift of your time and attention.

Concluding Thoughts

If you've done the exercises in this chapter, you've begun to create a safe place for the child that dwells within you. You've also identified and made a connection with whatever Spirit that child believes in. That core relationship is a crucial building block for future steps—because that is the place where we begin to knit back together. If the wound holds the answer, and the trauma creates the tools to heal from it, the connection between your inner child and Spirit generates the map for your pathway.

You may have noticed that those three concepts are very similar to each other. Each reflects a different paradox at the heart of any spiritual journey. If you've read any writings from the world's religions, you know that quest stories are full of paradoxes—we have to do what's hardest, let go of what we can't bear to release, face the fear that may kill us, and ask those who can't trust anyone to have faith. Your own route to healing will be just like this.

The rest of this work will require courage and strength. Luckily, you already have both—otherwise, you wouldn't be self-harming in the first place, and you certainly wouldn't be reading this book.

You're a warrior of the mind, bravely fighting the only enemy you can see. It's time to befriend that enemy and put that courage and strength to better use.

It also requires a belief that you can find your way to healing. It will take you through a tough portion of the path, one that every hero has to fight through, whether it's a forest of thorny branches, the land of Oz, an island of sirens, or the Death Star.

My inner Faith is going to show you the way.

"I said: what about my eyes?
He said: Keep them on the road.

I said: What about my passion:
He said: Keep it burning.

I said: What about my heart?
He said: Tell me what you hold inside it?

I said: Pain and sorrow.
He said: Stay with it. The wound is the place where the Light enters you."

—Rumi

"By the roots of my hair some god got hold of me. I sizzled in his blue volts like a desert prophet."

—Sylvia Plath,
from her poem *The Hanging Man*

CHAPTER FIVE

FAITH IN THE DARKNESS

One of my favorite places to hunt for answers was the old Bodhi Tree bookstore in Los Angeles. It just *smelled* of wisdom, with the incense and sitar music in the background. It was filled with books on ancient Eastern philosophies and modern interpretations. To my Western mind, these things symbolized mysterious teachings that would show me the way out of suffering. And I learned a lot from those books. It was the same with the yoga classes, the practice of kundalini, and meditating on my Vedic mantra, which I received from a guru who studied with the Maharishi Mahesh Yogi in India. Los Angeles, at the fulcrum of the millennium, was an amazing place to be if you were searching for truth—which I was always doing.

I researched human potential movements—Positive Psychology, Law of Attraction, A Course in Miracles—ideas that mined ancient wisdom from Stoicism, the Bhagavad Gita, Buddhism, Taoism, the Gnostic Gospels, and more. I followed different practitioners-turned-gurus promoting their personal brands of breath training, meditation, habit reform, time management, abundance creation, dietary plans, and every variety of regimes designed to help us live our best lives.

To this day, I meditate and pray every day. I eat well, exercise, and practice affirmations and breathing patterns. I use algorithms to program new habits, to refine my daily protocol, and maximize my potential. This book is being created during my regularly scheduled morning writing hours. And, of course, it's a direct result of my belief that our traumas can become our greatest strengths. Each foray contributed to my arsenal of tools. Each helped me climb steadily, slowly, out of the abyss and into the light.

And yet.

Every time I read a new book on how I could change with the right behavior or thinking pattern, part of me knocked on the door of my heart, sending melancholy echoes through my body.

It said, in a small voice, *What about me?*

No matter how much I learned, re-programmed, changed, and improved, the Cutter kept coming back. Willpower only kept it contained for so long. It was part of me and had nowhere else to go.

Have you felt anything like that? Perhaps you've overcome an addiction or changed a behavior, yet you secretly dread it will come back one day? It's as if there's a saboteur lurking inside, just out of reach, waiting for us to let our guard down so it can ambush us. In 12-step groups, people in recovery sometimes talk about their addict as a separate person who is outside the meeting room doing push-ups, getting stronger, waiting for that moment when they can take over again.

Somewhere along the way, that voice got so loud and overwhelming that I couldn't hear anything else. My effort to avoid it almost led me to relapse in alcohol and drugs. It landed me in an urgent care clinic with second-degree burns on my arm from self-injury—at forty-four years old.

I had to find a new way to view the Cutter—and the whole addict-doing-pushups story. Because that being lived inside me, not outside—it could take over without my permission or control. Just doing an inventory and turning it over to my higher power wasn't enough. Banishing my negative voices or outlawing negativity couldn't make it go away. Those were exercises, intellectual forays, not the actual battle.

One of my favorite inspiring anecdotes came from my friend Barb, who told me about the difference between the buffalo and the cow. Apparently, when a storm approaches, cows run in the opposite direction, trying to escape—which only prolongs their suffering, as the weather catches up and pummels them. But buffaloes walk toward it. Somehow, they figured out that if they lean in, the storm will pass faster.

So, I finally opened that locked door in my mind and met what I feared most—that part of me that I'd disowned.

It turned out to be what I'd been looking for all along.

My Experience

The first time I encountered the Cutter face-to-face, I had just started working with my new therapist. I was deep into the self-injury relapse. My partner was not happy about it—the behavior was frightening and threatening to her. Our relationship was fraying at the edges. Her mother had just died in our house, her father was soon to follow. Her parents' crises had added even more burdens to our stressed lives, and I felt tremendous pressure.

My therapist and I were working on grounding and safety in session that day. I wasn't expecting anything out of the ordinary when she simply asked me to become aware of what I was experiencing in my body. As I described the sensation in my chest, it suddenly exploded. Energy coursed through my interior. My teeth buzzed and my hands went numb. I could hardly breathe, and my heart was racing so fast. Later, she told me my face reddened and my pupils dilated. I thought I was going to shoot off through the ceiling. I sobbed as I struggled to control my body. The storm was upon me.

I sensed an amorphous tangle of darkness detach from my chest and hover outside, looking at me, held by a thread. Then it sucked back into me with a jolt.

My therapist instructed me to breathe, to feel the couch against my palms and the floor beneath my feet. It took some time to calm my chemistry. I felt unreal, far away—like I'd shot out of myself and couldn't get back inside. I could hardly talk about what had happened, but after I got home, I drew a picture. It surprised me to see it. This was the Cutter—I knew it. And yet it hadn't felt threatening. It was as confused as I was by this encounter.

Why were we attached by a string?

After this cathartic experience, I decided to throw away my blades. My therapist warned me that it might be too destabilizing to stop all at once—that the behavior served a vital purpose in my psyche, and I needed to unearth what was causing it before I could let it go. But I insisted. I stayed abstinent for three months—until a particularly tough argument with my partner, when I relapsed again, worse than before.

It took another few months for me to gather the strength to move out. It was the hardest thing I'd ever gone through in adulthood. I moved into a friend's daughter's old bedroom. There in that pink room looking onto an alley, I slid into the abyss.

For the next several months, while my partner and I tried and failed to patch things up, I cried my brains out. Sometimes I just lay on the floor and sobbed. Even the bed felt too far away. I floated on a turbulent sea like a straw in a hurricane. At my therapist's urging, I finally went to a psychiatrist. I refused all medications except for a half-dose of an SSRI (Selective Serotonin Reuptake Inhibitor), and after a few weeks, my suicidal ideation subsided, and I could breathe again. The work continued.

The Cutter began to appear more often during therapy. I had little control over the "surges." Once the energy burst through, my therapist would coach me through it, while I held on for dear life. Slowly, we both got to know this energy, or entity, as it became. She called it a dissociated part. I never "lost time"—which is what people with Dissociative Identity Disorder experience—but I definitely lost motor control. I could see myself from far away, just like I had when I used to cut myself, barely feeling pain.

I came to understand that this was a part of me—a disowned fragment that had no other way to communicate except through the dramatic act of self-harming. I acknowledged that it had always felt male—which was why it had never felt like *me* before, until that day it detached just enough to stare in my face. I couldn't deny that it dwelled inside me.

I remained committed to stopping self-harm—but it was slow, frustrating work. Paintings gave me a way to express what was going on inside, yet it sometimes felt dangerous to be alone in my art studio. Sometimes, I cut myself there. I'd promise to my therapist to abstain one day; the next, I couldn't even call her.

But the pauses in between grew longer. I told more people what I was going through so I could call upon other resources. I built my team. I gathered new tools.

One day, my therapist asked me what that part of me would say if he weren't cutting my skin. And so, I asked him to write it in red ink instead of blood.

He wrote "Help" on my upper arm. We began to have a dialogue.

I learned that he wasn't a supernatural male spirit after all—he was my young tomboy, the one who had endured the sexual abuse and buried it in a secret place inside. He didn't want to be a girl because bad things happened to girls. His rage was huge. It protected us from harm. But at the same time, he was trapped in a dungeon, and I had to let him out. He'd saved our life; he needed me to save his.

Just calling him "Maggie" didn't feel right. After all, he'd existed in a world of his own for years. When I asked him what he should be called, he gave me his name. It was *Faith*.

After that, everything fell into place. Faith was the one who visited the dragon—his protector, his ally. Faith was also the one who guarded our treasure, who slashed the dummy when he got mad.

Slowly, we learned to trust each other. I got a "Faith" tattoo on the spot where we'd written "Help." While the needle was pressing ink into my skin, Faith and I worked together to numb the pain, with a clear understanding that it was for good, not self-harm.

Once in therapy, as Faith was coursing through me, my therapist gave me a pen and paper—and I observed myself furiously scribbling, not lifting the pen, until I poked through the paper. Afterward, I stared at the image, incredulous that it had come from me. Faith had written words that he then covered over. That was how he protected the secret. But I saw it; my therapist saw it. A message had been sent and received.

After that, I got a special journal and let him draw whenever he wanted. His work was spontaneous, aggressive. It was like cutting with a pen—except the paper received the lines instead of my skin. He kept writing words then scribbling over them. The main thing he kept saying, in one way or another, was *It Did Happen*.

I put pieces together and realized that the cutting was linked to the unfair punishments I received growing up. If I left the dish on the wrong side of the sink, or locked a door, or sucked my thumb, Dad told me what happened next was my fault—so I believed I deserved the abuse. I learned to identify it as gaslighting—that insidious blame-the-victim strategy all abusers employ. That dynamic played out in all my adult relationships—including the one with my own inner child. I didn't know any other way to parent except to set up impossible rules, then beat myself up when I broke them. Or get someone else to do it for me.

Eventually, Faith was able to illustrate the sexual abuse. To this day, I've never been able to say the words out loud, but Faith can share the images with his pen.

Stopping the self-injury happened on its own, as I learned to listen to what Faith had been trying to say all along. *Pay attention to me, believe me, rescue me, love me.*

I stopped questioning that the abuse happened. I stopped beating myself up. I let go of people who treated me the way I'd been taught to expect. I started listening to my internal parts, to my body's needs, and practicing better self-care. I began to love myself.

All of this required trust (faith), a loving guide, a willingness to embrace what was happening, and time. It wasn't easy to stop the behavior of cutting, even after befriending Faith. The behavior had an addictive pull that was hard to shake. But I made commitments, told more people, painted a lot, worked my recovery program, and explored my interior. I gave my therapist my last "active" blade. She kept it in my file for a long time, until I was ready for her to discard it. The chemistry fueling my self-harm subsided. I cemented new pathways in my brain.

The entire process of relapsing to recovery took about six years. A whole lifetime passed during that time. Faith wasn't the only part

I encountered in my fragmented interior—he was the gatekeeper who allowed others to emerge. Folding him back into me freed a tremendous amount of energy. It gave me a story of my interior that finally made sense, that connected me to *me*.

After that initial recovery phase, it took me another six years of settling into myself to become ready to share this story with others. What at first seemed odd, doubtful, and embarrassing is now my truth—and I don't need to question it anymore. Faith is more real to me than this chair I'm sitting on as I type.

Now, he's an essential part of me. He speaks up, he paints the internal storm, and he is our strength. I take care of him. When I sense a surge bubbling up, I check inside and ask him what's going on. It took time to establish a mutually trusting relationship, but now he tells me right away when he's upset. I try my best to take good care of him. I give him the stage when he needs to talk. We are a family now.

Faith taught me another paradox: *The only way around the problem is to go right through it.* Faith was the one I'd been avoiding all those years, but he's the one I needed to help me move on toward healing. The one who trusted no one had to embody faith in order to survive.

The wound held the answer.

Your Experience

Now is the time to clarify what I mean when I talk about *stopping* self-harm. This is not about taking a solemn vow—that's a set-up for disappointment and self-flagellation. Willpower alone is not enough. If it were, we would have stopped every time someone asked us to.

The physical craving for the chemical high takes a while to release. In 12-step programs, addicts surrender in order to get power back. They *decide* to turn their lives over to Spirit (a God of their understanding), then Spirit does the work of removing their addictions and changing their lives.

It's the same with cutting. The mechanics of the addiction may differ, but the process is the same. It requires a willingness to trust that if we do the work, the obsession will be removed. It requires faith in a future we can't see. But we're searching for that Spirit or higher power *inside us*, not up in the sky. We look inward for the answers, not outward. Instead of demonizing the addiction, we view it as a form of communication, a voice on the skin. And we approach it with compassion.

We give the self-harming part different prompts. *What are you trying to say? Where do you live inside? What do you need from me now?*

I suggest you work with your therapist to come up with a way to communicate regularly with that part of you. If you do slip and self-harm, instead of berating yourself, try the opposite approach. Thank yourself for refusing to stay silent. Be gentle with your wound as you would with your own child or pet. Ask the one who injures if they could try another way of getting your attention next time—and promise that you will listen better.

This is the work of the buffalo. Everything has led up to this—meeting and embracing the disowned part that is injuring the body. That is the one you've been looking for all along.

Peter Levine put it best when he said:

> Trauma is the fourth pathway to awakening. In transforming and releasing ourselves from trauma we must face, as does the newborn child, an

uncertain world. It is a world stripped of the illusion of safety, and it obliges us to learn an entirely new way of being. When we enter it, we soon discover that our instinctive energies are not limited to acts of flight or uncontrolled violence. They are our *heroic energies*. And they can be harnessed! The energies that are released when we heal from trauma are the wellspring of our creative, artistic, and poetic sensibilities, and they can be summoned to propel us into the wholeness of our intelligence.[15]

Let's unlock the doors to those ancient cells inside us. Creativity is the way in—the part that is waiting for you will lead the way.

Grounding Technique: Box Breathing

Breathing exercises have been shown to regulate stress, metabolism, mood, sleep, and so much more. Just the simple act of breathing through the nose brings calm. If we breathe into the belly more than the chest, that carries it even further.

Structured *pranayama*, or breath work, originated in India as a discipline of yoga. U.S. Navy SEALs adopted some of those techniques to help soldiers maintain calm in the midst of battle. The most famous of these, box breathing, is also used by first responders, professional athletes, and others who need to calm their nerves to perform in stressful situations.

This is a good technique to use whenever you feel overwhelmed. Whatever trauma initiated the impulse to self-harm has left a residue of adrenaline inside our bodies—and it can get randomly released at unexpected times. It can make us feel like something

---

[15] Levine, *Healing Trauma*, 90-91.

terrible and dangerous is happening *right now*. When that occurs, it's important to calm the body before anything else.

The method is easy. Just breathe in for a count of four, hold for four, then out for four, hold for four. It's best to do it with your eyes closed, if you feel safe doing so, and to breathe through the nose. When you hold the breath in or out, do it gently, without straining. The four-count can go at any pace that feels comfortable. Concentrate on centering, soothing, and letting go. Breathe into the belly more. Slow down the pace of the count.

If the mind is panicking about external threats, it might help to re-imagine that plexiglass box from chapter two. As you breathe in, walk along one of those walls to the corner and check its strength. Hold the breath and walk to the next wall, check the corner, exhale along the third wall, and hold it out as you complete the square. Meditate on the integrity of this protective membrane as you slow down the count. You'll know you're done by how it feels inside.

This is a powerful breathing technique and can be practiced every day to cultivate overall calm. If Navy SEALs do it to prepare for battle situations, we can use it to face inner chaos.

Before trying any of the exercises below, I want to reiterate the importance of body grounding. In chapter four, we went over specific exercises like butterfly tapping and mindfulness. You might want to write something like "butterfly tapping" or "check all five senses" on a piece of paper that you keep nearby to remind you what to do if you dissociate. Or you might put your talisman, drawing of Spirit, or Sculpey figure next to you so you can see it or hold onto it when you get lost.

If you're anything like me, you're probably impatient to engage in the process as deeply and quickly as possible to get through it faster—but it's not something that can be rushed with willpower.

Like a farmer yanking on the new shoots to make them grow faster, you'll just upset the natural flow of development.

Remember, the fastest way is to go slow.

Visualization: Faith in the Body

Sit in a comfortable place with your journal and pen next to you. Close your eyes. Pay attention to your breathing. Follow the breath as it moves through your lungs and down into your belly. Feel it flow out as you exhale. Scan your body for any places where you feel stuck or hurt. There might be a spot that is numb or blank. Note where you feel good. There's no need to fix anything, just observe.

Now, focus on the site where you last self-harmed. Feel energy inside that wound or scar. Picture yourself in the midst of the act. Don't be afraid—this is only happening inside your mind, nowhere else. You have the power to experience that part and to observe it at the same time. Push deeper into that feeling. Let yourself become it. Note any physiological changes from the inside. Keep breathing. Open your mind into a state of curiosity and see what comes to you.

Sit up taller, extend your neck, and lift your chin. Let yourself feel power. Allow pride to course through. Note any images or sounds that arise.

Does that part have a symbol or spirit of their own? Do they have a name? Thank them for being so persistent in their communication and for refusing to back down. If tears come, let the emotion storm through and out.

The first time you connect with the entity or energy that self-harms, it may feel overwhelming. Then again, your connection might be blissful or relieving. Let it flow through you without resistance. Trust that it will pass. Perhaps you could repeat the word *faith* to guide you through.

When the energy has subsided, focus back on your breathing. Count the inhale, hold at the top, then exhale for a longer count. Do that a few times. Then open your eyes.

Turn to your journal and describe or draw what you saw. Perhaps it was just a vague energy. Perhaps it was some concrete being or part. Does it have a gender? Did it give you a name? Can you see it as part of you? How does it make you feel?

If you feel overstimulated by the experience, do some butterfly tapping. Go for a walk or drink a glass of water. Congratulate yourself for having the courage to do this. It can be very strange to encounter new parts of ourselves. They're not really new—they've just been hidden from our conscious awareness by our brilliant mechanisms of self-protection. They belong to us—and there's no reason to feel scared or embarrassed. We have every right to claim the terrain of our own interior.

Exercise: Let Your Skin Talk

You'll need a red pen and your journal or a larger piece of paper. It's probably best not to use a Sharpie, and stay away from the ballpoint pens. This is an exercise in healing, not harming.

If you've typically self-harmed in front of the mirror, take your place there. Look fully at your own reflection while you do this exercise.

When you pick up the pen to write or draw, describe, out loud, its color, its weight, how it feels on your fingers, and what sound it makes as it scratches against paper. Smell the ink. Become aware of your eyes seeing it, your hand holding it, your seat in the chair, and your feet on the floor. Note your presence in the room.

Choose the place on your skin that you usually injure or are thinking about injuring. Close your eyes and focus your attention there. Feel the energy that you channeled in the visualization above. If it has a name, call it forth. Invite it to come in and sit next to you. Allow the presence to linger without reactiveness. Ask what it/he/she/they are trying to say.

Open your eyes now and write that answer on your skin. It might be a phrase, picture, or symbol. If your internal part wants to draw on another part of you, let them.

If you feel resistance or embarrassment, let it flow through and away. Allow yourself to take this seriously. So often, we censor ourselves for fear of what people might think or whether they will shame us over being different or "crazy."

But which is preferable, a bleeding wound or a word scrawled in red ink?

Another option is to get a doll that represents you or a childhood plush toy. Or you could make something with Sculpey or some other materials. It helps if it's three-dimensional rather than just a flat drawing. Follow the instructions above, then use that red pen to mark on the doll's arm (or other body part).

Whatever method you use, take a picture of the marking. That helps cement the communication, giving it permanence after the ink is washed away. Keep that photo handy for the next time you feel an urge to self-harm. Remain curious about the message it's giving you. When you're ready, share it with someone you trust. You're stepping out of the bounds of silence, honoring the voice on your skin.

Exercise: Rage Art

Although the act of cutting might seem calm and controlled, it's actually expressing anger—not just anger, but seething rage, along with tidal waves of despair, grief, and terror. A lot of intense energy is being distilled into that act. Some of us harbor a fear that if we let it loose in some other way, it would detonate our entire world.

It might feel like an explosion, but it's just feelings, not real destruction. Having said that, it's important to have a steady hand to guide us through. Before embarking on these next few exercises, please share with your therapist or guide that you'll be engaging with big emotions. The ultimate goal is to voice them in a healthy, contained way, but if at any point it triggers more self-harming, this may not be the time. Talk with your therapist and review your tools. Make a plan to self-soothe after each exercise.

First, we're going to try some "rage art." That's what I called the drawings Faith did. From the outside, it looks like automatic scribbling. From the inside, it's an experience of letting the feelings do the talking.

The choice of when to do this exercise is very personal. For me, I did it after I felt triggered by something. After working on it in therapy for so many years, I could recognize the signs of a growing urge. It was physiological as well as mental and emotional. It gathered energy as it continued—so I began to do the rage art to re-direct that build-up. In other words, I drew when I felt overwhelmed—but before it reached the point of no return. The rage art became one of those "instead of" tools, not to be used lightly—kind of a "big gun" in my arsenal.

If you have a playlist or other sensory item that accompanied your self-harming before, try adding that to the creative session. Be cautious about overwhelming your system with triggers.

The setup for this exercise is simple. Open your journal and tune into the feelings that trigger self-harming. But instead of picking up a blade, pick up your pen and start to draw. Resolve to maintain contact with the page. Draw and write and scribble all those feelings and thoughts. Let yourself get mad and overwhelmed.

Get it all out. Your eyes might close halfway. You might embody the feelings with your posture. The important thing is to emote with your pen until it passes through you and away.

Afterward, stand up and stretch, drink some water or hot tea, take a bath, walk, or nap. Be gentle. Thank that part of you that communicated through a pen instead of a blade (or other mode of self-harm). Honor your courage. Work to calm down the chemistry.

Another exercise is to Smash the Noise. I encountered versions of this in various workshops I attended over the years, and I adapted it for my use. This is also meant to replace the act of self-harming. Its purpose is to interrupt (and re-groove) the old pathway from trigger to action. By saving this type of exercise for the times when the adrenaline is high and the urge is strong, we preserve its potency.

Many of us have critical voices in our heads. It's hard to hear anything else amidst a chorus of mocking, berating, hateful thoughts. It took me a long time to separate those from the actual voice of my Cutter (Faith), who was trying to slip a note through the bars. Those critics are the gatekeepers who want to silence the child's voice. In the Internal Family Systems (IFS) model, they're seen as Managers and Firefighters.[16]

They are the warnings we learned from caregivers who couldn't bear to hear our truth, and they've been honed into weapons of mass destruction through years of repetition. A lot of people have shared what their critical voices have said with me, and they all say some version of the same thing. *You're not worthy. You're unlovable. You're lying. You're stupid. Be quiet.*

Write down what they say—every word. Fill a whole page with those nasty messages—all the things you say to yourself in the privacy of your own head. Don't hold back.

---

[16] Schwartz, *No Bad Parts*, 73–74.

When you've vented all the meanness, separate the messages, by cutting them out or tearing them into pieces. Now get a thick pillow or patio cushion and cover it with an old pillowcase. Get a hammer or mallet. Find a private place where you won't be disturbed. Pile those pieces of hate onto the pillow and smash the hell out of each one. Put all your energy into that arm. Obliterate every word, one by one. Either mentally or out loud, tell those voices you aren't going to listen anymore. They don't have the power to silence you. It's time for you to speak up. Get loud!

Afterward, look at the shreds of what you destroyed. Are they beaten to a pulp? Can you still see words? How does it feel to see them torn apart? Can you thank these fearful messages and appreciate that they once protected you?

You can either burn these vestiges, or you can save them for a future exercise. The hammer or mallet you just used is your new tool. It's a portal to the pent-up energy inside. You might want to honor it in some way by decorating it or storing it in a special place. I used a black Sharpie to "tattoo" the neck of my mallet. It became my secret weapon against the old lies.

There are other ways to vent that energy. Some cities have "smash rooms" that give customers an opportunity to break things at will. If you live in the country, you might find some old windows and shatter them with a baseball bat or throw broken dishes at a wall. The important thing is to do it safely and with intention, knowing who you're channeling and why—then finish up with self-soothing and a message of thanks to your internal world. Just stirring up anger for its own sake may be more harmful than healing, so you'll want to do it as part of a larger plan with your therapist or guide.

The internal parts that have caused us so much trouble are not going away. They are part of us. We can no more get rid of them than we can cut off our own arm. We have to befriend them, let them vent feelings and messages, and then fold them back in with love.

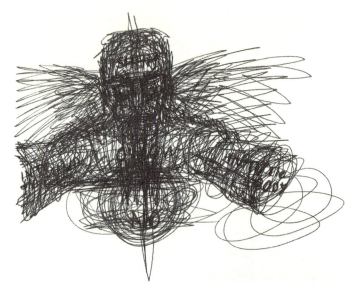

Figure 8: One of Faith's early drawings, done in ink without lifting the pen. He often wrote phrases about the abuse, then scribbled over to hide the words.

Exercise: Tactile Substitutes

When I was about seven or eight, one of my mother's art students melted army men and made them into pins as statements about nuclear weapons. I didn't understand the politics of his work—I just wanted to try it for myself. So, I gathered all my plastic army men and figurines, took them outside with a lighter, and burned them into nubs.

Perhaps another parent might have been worried, but my mother was amused by my attempts at making art. I was more interested in watching the soldiers' weapons and arms curl up as they melted.

My childhood drawings were full of people battling monsters, or each other. In real life, I was fighting everyone I knew, mostly boys, especially if they were bigger and could kick the crap out of me. Being able to vent feelings with creativity directed my anger into something less harmful to myself and others, if only for a short time.

I won't officially advocate burning plastic or encourage you to use a lighter—but if you choose to try something like this for yourself, the details are up to you. Find/buy/create a figurine or doll that you can destroy. It could represent a negative force or abuser that you wish to annihilate, or it could be a stand-in for your inner hater (which is really an avatar for the crap that others piled on you).

Decorate it with the hater's mean words—or cover it with the pieces of paper from the earlier exercise. Tell it, out loud, that you don't accept their lies anymore.

Then destroy it. Creatively. Banish those words forever. Get physical, release the energy. Don't feel bad for that figurine—it's just an emotionless doll. Lies are empty, weak, ephemeral. They only have power if we grant it to them.

When you're done, you can decide what to do with the remains of that negativity. Burn it, bury it, throw it in the trash. Take some deep breaths and send it on its way.

Every time you hear that voice again, remind yourself it's just a ghost, it's not real. The truth is that you are worthy, lovable, capable, and strong. You didn't deserve to be hurt. You're in charge now. And unless that lie wants to be pounded, cut, and burned again, they'd better get the hell away.

Exercise: The Warrior's Story

All of this creative expression is helping you tell a new story. The characters and plot are up to you. Somewhere in this chaotic emoting, a narrative will emerge. Perhaps, like I did, you've encountered the one inside who did the harming. Or maybe you're just getting out your feelings. Whatever is coming out belongs to you, and it wants your attention.

I was always trying to paint my Cutter. For years, it was a mystical being who dwelled outside of me, waiting to come in and take over. That strange conundrum occupied most of my artistic forays. Once I found Faith, I let him do the creating. I located him inside and gave him a voice. Faith is the one who creates my most energetic work. He's the one who has the courage to risk destroying a painting in order to push it through to its completion.

So, why don't you try drawing the one inside you who feels so stuck that the only way for them to be okay is to harm your body?

It doesn't matter if you're an artist or not. You can write about it if you prefer, but something about creating a visual representation, however crude, makes the abstract more concrete. This being inside you is not a literal person—so it can look like anything.

Just put pen to paper with the intention of drawing something that represents it, and you will get a result, I promise. Let it flow from your pen.

When you're done, look at what came out. Get curious about it. How old is it? Is it human, animal, or angel? Who is its higher power? What is it wearing if anything? Did it share its name? Draw those things. Write them down.

Don't be frightened by its blustering and threats. This part of you had to get very big to keep your life force intact—but ultimately, *its entire purpose is to protect you*. Anger in itself is a healthy emotion, one that every human being experiences. We just never learned how to express it in healthy ways. Whatever moved you to push a sharp or hot object against your skin, or stick a finger down your throat, or tear your hair can actually be harnessed and turned into a strength. It's a vital part of you. It's time to reclaim it.

If you want to take this further, you could create a comic about this part. Or you could let the part tell *you* their story through a comic. Let the kid inside draw it. Using simple figures and dialog bubbles, let that part tell you what they went through, where they live now, and what they're trying to do with the self-harming. Take time to read what they create and thank them for sharing it with you.

When I was getting to know Faith, I created a comic bearing his name, about a transgender superhero fighting hate crimes. The entire narrative came through me in a flash—then it took me years to develop it into a graphic novel series. I never got it published, but it taught me a lot about finding self-acceptance in a violent world.

Like I've said before, we cannot erase that internal part that harms us. I tried banishing it many times, only to have it boomerang back stronger than ever. I didn't find true liberation until I finally turned around to face it and fold it back into me. It *was* me.

The voice on your skin isn't trying to get the whole world to listen—it's trying to get *you* to listen. You're the only one who will truly understand what they're trying to say.

Exercise: Kali Art

In many Hindu traditions, the goddess Kali is feared and revered. A powerful entity, she is a frightening destroyer who is often depicted with charcoal black skin, wearing a necklace of skulls, a skirt of severed hands, and other evidence of bloody mayhem. One of many forms of the Shakti, goddess Kali is the one who blasts out obstacles so that new gifts can emerge. She grants boons to those who please her.

Long before I learned about Kali, I'd incorporated this energy into my own art-making process. It started with a fiber arts class in college. Our professor taught us how to dye silk, and the results were beautiful. We students politely critiqued each other's work as directed, but secretly felt all the pieces were so nice they didn't need changing. However, our teacher had other ideas. She directed us to destroy our pieces and transform them into something new, using any of the collaging materials in the studio, and whatever space we chose. After swallowing our disappointment that these lovely silks could only exist for a short amount of time, we each went on to create amazing works of art. One young man cut his orange-dyed silk into flame shapes, which he stiffened with wax, then hung from a line so he could burn it in a ceremonial fire. I cut my blue-green tapestry into fish shapes, which I hid in the bushes around the studio. We each let go of the "precious-ness" of the pieces in order to mold them into mature works of art.

That lesson has stayed with me. When I first tried to stop self-harming in sobriety, I gave the Cutter (who hadn't told me his name yet) a healthier job. He became the one who "destroyed" a piece to create something else. He's the one who decided one day to completely paint over an image (which I'd started to like too much) with ultramarine. Mortified, I tried to wipe that off with a rag soaked in mineral oil spirits (paint remover). It was too late—the pigment had stained it too much. But as I rubbed it away, the underlayer emerged in unexpected shapes, like haunting, blue ghosts—leading to a much better image in the end.

That turned into an essential part of my painting practice. Once I fall in love with an artwork, I cover it with a counter-intuitive coat of color, or I wipe off the whole layer with textured rags. It's scary at first because I have no idea if that will ruin the piece, but it always turns out to be the key to reaching the final image.

Faith taught me that I have to let go of my attachment to where I *think* the piece going in order to discover where it's *supposed* to go. I have to risk destroying it to break through to the final creation. I have to listen to what the painting is trying to say. I employ Kali energy to bring out the real gift of the work.

So, try that in your own art. Either take one of the pieces you've done in these exercises, or something you've done on your own, and destroy it in some way. If it's on paper, try cutting it into pieces and make a collage, then paint on top. If it's a painting, cover it with a layer of paint in a color that disturbs you, then slowly remove parts of it, letting a new composition emerge. Remember that exercise where you colored different squares? Take out a black pencil and start coloring over them—lightly at first, then harder when you want to blacken out areas. Enjoy the subtle new colors that are created in the process.

If you're a sculptor or ceramicist, break a piece and seam it back together, or create an entirely new figure with the shards. If you've been knitting something, shred or cut it into pieces then shape it into a three-dimensional figure with wires, string, or twigs. See if you can maintain that powerful destructive energy as you reassemble it into something new.

You could also try "blackout poetry," a form of redacting an existing piece to reveal a hidden poem. It's usually done by crossing out lines of an existing piece, like an essay or article, leaving select words or phrases intact. The remaining fragments become a haphazard poem. It can hold layers of meaning, depending on which sections are left open and which piece was chosen for the exercise. I tried this with a page of one of my father's letters and came up with something that not only read as a completely different piece, but also changed the energy in his words.

Feel the energy that is harnessed when you allow yourself to destroy then re-create. The part of you that self-harmed is quite powerful—and it can become an important part of you to be called upon when needed. Practice that in your creative work. Bring the strongest parts of you into your artmaking.

As Jesus said in the Gnostic Gospel of Thomas, "If you bring forth what is within you, what you bring forth will save you; if you do not bring forth what is within you, what you do not bring forth will destroy you."

So, bring it forth!

Advanced Exercises: Energize the Work

Many artists throughout time have incorporated physical gestures in their work. Jackson Pollock, often credited for popularizing Abstract Expressionism, hurled globs of paint across huge canvases on the floor. I was once commissioned to do a Pollock-style portrait of Mickey Mouse for Imagineering, and I discovered that it's very therapeutic to get sloppy and aggressive with paint. I still had to maintain a semblance of a character underneath, but it was fun to see how far I could take it. I think everyone should do a Pollock-style drip painting at some point in their career.

If you want to try it, lay a canvas across the floor, or tack it on a wall—wherever you can get sloppy. Dip your brush into red paint and splatter it. Let the physical gesture express what you've been trying to say. You can even swear while you're splattering. It doesn't matter what it looks like—just let your internal part (or parts) create to their heart's content.

Have you ever tried to paint your emotions? Not a strict portrait, but an expression? What does it *feel* like to self-harm? Who is feeling it inside? Paint them. Who are you mad at? Paint them. What is the energy like? Is it explosive, quiet, fiery, or cold? Are there shards, blades, or mushroom clouds? Is there a shape inside all that? Are there words?

As I've mentioned, I used to add cuts into my paintings. I'd add a layer of gesso onto a canvas and use a blade that might otherwise be used for cutting to slash lines into it. Then after it dried, I'd drip red paint into the grooves. It wasn't just a random act, it was intentional. I'd play the music I used to listen to while cutting and slip into a trance as I created. I summoned the Cutter and gave it a new task. An intense painting session would leave me feeling cleaned out, the way self-harming used to do, except I was also proud that I'd created something beautiful instead of a new wound on my skin.

If you want to try this, all you need is a canvas, acrylic gesso, a brush, and a blade. Brush a thick layer of gesso onto the canvas. Let it dry a little, then run the sharp edge lightly through its doughy skin. Don't dig so deep that it damages the substrate underneath. Try imitating the pattern you use when self-harming. When it dries, add red paint into the grooves. Let those marks grow into a larger image. Let it express what the self-harming is trying to say.

What image comes out? Can you turn it into a self-portrait? How do the "cuts" influence the larger form? Who is that person who cuts, and what do they look like? Can you transform those lines into swords, or arrows? Or musculature, veins, or bones?

If nothing comes to mind, try the Listening Doodle from chapter one—let a line tell you what it needs next, then paint that in. Respond to the shape it creates by enhancing it. Slip into a more unconscious state of painting around the red lines. This doesn't need to be a masterpiece—it's just a way of dialoguing with the one who self-harms.

Remember, feelings are not lethal—only their repression creates ill health. Creative gestures are the safest way to "off-gas" long-suppressed emotions.

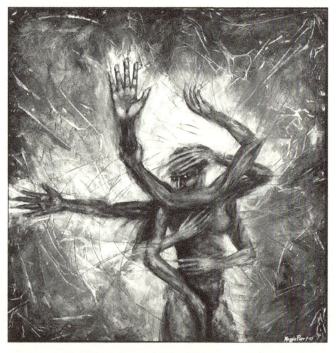

Figure 9: "The Confrontation," Oil on canvas, 1997. A visceral response to writing my father a confrontation letter.

Reflection

Creativity is your way into the parts of you that are frozen or lost, and creativity is how you build new pathways in thinking and behavior. It loosens the grip of your restrictive voices of judgment, fear, and criticism.

Journal about what you experienced in this chapter. Document what's happening. Organize it into stories that make sense to you.

Does your self-harming part have a name? Can you see them, feel their presence inside you? What have they been trying to tell you? Is trust building between you?

If none of this made sense, or you feel overwhelmed, can you find a spark of reality, truth, or stability inside?

Take some time to list out the gains you've made so far. It's so easy to get discouraged, exhausted, and lose hope. But progress has been made. Look at how brave you are. Your therapist or guide can remind you how far you've come. Everything becomes more real, more powerful, with the affirmation of a compassionate witness.

Concluding Thoughts

Having carried us through the hardest part of the work, Faith says, "Do you see now?" He's eager to explain what's so important about doing this work—it's the way back in! And it's not that scary after all. Once you shine a light into all the dark crannies, the shadows don't loom so large. It's not a monster in that corner, it's an ancient rock that looks like a monster. When you turn the light on, it doesn't look scary at all.

There's no turning back now. The only way around the pain is by going right through the middle of it.

It was such a revelation for me to realize that Faith (the Cutter) wasn't trying to hurt me, he was trying to get my attention. He came into being because he was protecting someone—the little girl who was being abused. Faith had to get big and loud to try and get help. He spent the next forty years knocking at the door of my skin, trying to get me to rescue that innocent part that had long been asleep, waiting until it was safe enough to come out.

A lot of life happened in those forty years. I had to reenact my family of origin dynamics many times until I finally learned how not to. Then, I had to build a safe place of my own to do this work.

My hope for you is that you find a way to befriend your own hurt kid inside—the one who is cutting as a way to get what they need. These exercises will help, or they may give you ideas for creating your own. You may or may not have breakthroughs. Be patient. Just starting the work creates the next steps in the path, which has a tempo of its own and is unique to you. It's not easy or quick.

Celebrate your progress, however small. You're already in the hardest part—it gets easier from here. We may visit the abyss, but it will never be as frightening, because we've become familiar with the terrain. By lifting the stone from the buried chaos, we release tremendous energy—and we can leverage it to release more energy. Every little victory becomes a new weapon for change, and it connects us to others who have suffered—which is virtually everyone.

It's time to take a break from the heaviness and meet the one we've been protecting all along.

'Hope' Is the Thing with Feathers

"Hope" is the thing with feathers –
That perches in the soul –
And sings the tune without the words –
And never stops – at all –

And sweetest – in the Gale – is heard –
And sore must be the storm –
That could abash the little Bird
That kept so many warm –

I've heard it in the chillest land –
And on the strangest Sea –
Yet – never – in Extremity,
It asked a crumb – of me.

—Emily Dickinson

CHAPTER SIX

HOPE IS THE GLUE

To help me find balance in my inner work, my therapist gave me an illustration of an infinity sign. She traced the sideways eight shape and described how one side is the heavy work of grief, and the other side is the lighter distractions—reading, spending time outdoors, seeing movies, laughing, and so on. We loop around in one area, then we traverse the line and spend some time on the opposite side, never spending too long in one place.

In other words, we need balance. For those of us who can't predict or control when the darkness will rise up, that feels impossible. Self-harming is a way of avoiding pain—but the addictive habit keeps pain alive and well. Paradoxically, diving into it directly—but with intention, guidance, and tools—breaks the chains of addiction and allows us more choices.

So, it's time to exercise the muscle of *choosing* how to feel. We learn we can titrate back and forth from pain to joy, consciously acknowledging the benefits of both and allowing ourselves to feel the full range of emotions. The easiest way to do this is to practice having fun.

If it seems difficult at first, repetition will make it easier. Every time we see a break in the clouds, we can leverage it. If you had a good night's sleep and feel more hopeful, use that extra bit of energy to call a friend. If you've just exercised and feel stronger, eat something healthy and go to bed early. The sadness will return, but instead of seeing it as a failure, or a sign that it will never go away, accept that you're cycling through the infinity sign.

Scheduling a daily time for intentional recovery work will also help contain the feelings. If we know that at a certain time, we'll be sitting down to do some rage art, that makes it easier to stay present the rest of the day. Our internal parts begin to trust that each will get "airtime," that no difficulties will last forever. The messages are being sent and heard. Slowly, through practice and establishing new habits, the internal chemistry starts to settle.

Take comfort in knowing that the hardest part is over. Even if you're still in the thick of it, dealing with the aftereffects of trauma, struggling to stop self-harming, or stuck in depression, being *in* it is preferable to avoiding it. So much of addiction is trying to avoid feeling bad. Well, if you're feeling bad, you're experiencing the thing you've always feared—and if it hasn't killed you yet, then there's hope that things will get better.

As Thomas Merton said, "What you fear is an indication of what you seek." Keep turning toward the thing you've avoided, and eventually, it will cease to cause fear. It might even turn into a friend.

My Experience

I mentioned that Faith was protecting someone—well, it gradually became clear that what he was protecting was another part inside.

This part wasn't like Faith. It didn't take over with a rush of energy. It was a quiet, distant presence lying just beyond his shields. When Faith began to calm down and settle into me, the veil lifted, and there she was.

She appeared in one of my meditations as a little child in a bee costume, flying around my head. Her joy was infectious. She loved ladybugs, butterflies, orange trees, and lavender flowers. Through her eyes, I saw things I hadn't noticed before. She was the most innocent, happy part of me—the one who felt at home in the world. Mom used to tell me that when she took me on walks when I was little, it took forever because I had to stop and study every single thing along the way. Well, that kid was still there. Her untarnished love of the world began seeping into my adult consciousness. We woke up together.

I realized she needed a name, too, so I went inside and asked her what she'd like to be called. The answer was immediate. *My name is Hope.*

Hope connected deeply with my dear cat, Shilo. When I'd left my house of seventeen years, I'd accepted my partner's decree that I could not have any of our ten cats. But after we finally broke up, Shilo ran away, and didn't return. We assumed he was dead. Three and a half months later, on Valentine's Day, I got a call from a local shelter, miles away from my old home, telling me that he'd been found. My ex graciously agreed to let me have him (even though I was prepared to fight for him). After all that time on the streets, Shilo weighed only five pounds and was covered in fleas. I gave him baths and nursed him back to health. He nursed me back to health, too, as I was deep in my abyss. We healed each other. He was truly a miracle.

As Hope came alive, so did my paintings of Disney characters. My work with Imagineering had evolved to include more character work, mostly in murals and portraits. Before connecting with Hope inside, I'd sometimes struggled to connect with the cheerful imagery of the happiest place on earth. I often had to play horror movies in the background while I worked, just to balance it out. But with Hope running the show, I started to enjoy painting mice and ducks. I found an ease with the brush that allowed Spirit to flow through. My two styles of art—commercial and expressionist—didn't seem so far apart anymore. Playfulness entered my own paintings. I started listening to different music while I worked—less triggering, more inspirational. I de-rusted, sanded, and painted vintage tools and called the series "Spirit Tools."

Through my daily check-ins, these two child parts showed me their world. Faith told me that when things got rough, he put Hope to sleep to keep her safe, then he endured the abuse. He was constantly afraid that he wouldn't be up to the task. Sometimes he resented her—she got to sleep while he fought a losing battle—but mostly, he felt loyal to her, to his role as a warrior.

Hope let me know that she sleeps inside the tree—that place we'd visited in our early visualizations. Now it made sense why that was the first stop of my inner travels. Hope was the beginning of me. Her safe haven is a cozy interior with a small, soft bed. Baby animals of every kind join her there. Once all have entered, the trunk closes behind so no one else can enter without permission.

At first, Hope seemed ignorant to the abuse, but as time went on, she revealed that she'd agreed to go dormant in order to stay alive—but she saw what happened and understood what it meant. She carried a deep grief in her soul for what she'd lost—her trust in the world, her sense of safety, and her innocence. She'd lost faith and love. But with that grief came wisdom of a more existential kind. Hope was new enough in the world to still be connected to Spirit, and because of this, she saw the bigger picture of loss. Her sorrow joined the great chorus of human tears over the impermanence of life, security, joy, and happiness—the loss of innocence and the opportunity to love.

The sadness didn't stop her from delighting in the world's gifts. Just as she had when our body was tiny, she loved taking walks in this adult body. Every rock, every bug, every leaf had a spirit of its own that spoke to her in a secret language. We stopped to smell roses. We squatted down to move a caterpillar from the sidewalk into the grass.

In the past, whenever Faith got agitated, that was Hope's signal to go to sleep. But once she understood that she didn't have to disappear to stay alive, she could stay awake and help me soothe Faith. She thanked him for doing the hard work of fighting off the abuse.

Over time, her energy and insights trickled into my body and consciousness. Happiness appeared more often. I didn't question whether it would suddenly disappear, like a rug being yanked out from beneath my feet. I trusted it would stay.

I realized that I *felt* new hope and faith. Hope dwelled *within* Faith, like a nesting doll. By reconnecting with them, I'd plugged back into a deep source of power within me, and the gaping hole inside was filling back up.

My art became less trauma-focused and more joyful. Poetry had always inspired my painting, but when Hope came alive in me, I turned from the despairing voices of Emily Dickinson, John Donne, Sylvia Plath, and Anne Sexton toward more hopeful voices, like Mary Oliver, John O'Donohue, Pablo Neruda, and Kay Ryan. I printed out poems that held special weight and kept them in my purse for emergencies—like a first aid kit for existential wounds.

The act of cutting used to have a particular soundtrack— atmospheric, repetitive, haunting. I stopped listening to those songs during painting sessions, except for my favorites, like "Blue Lagoon" by Laurie Anderson. Painting with Hope called for a new soundtrack that was light, gentle, even happy. She danced to Beyoncé, Mary J. Blige, and Michael Franti. She made me play and replay Neil Young's "I Am a Child," "Man on Fire" by Edward Sharpe and the Magnetic Zeros, and "I Was a Bird" by Mary Chapin Carpenter. We always close our painting with Beethoven's "Ode to Joy."

She's the one who insisted we start painting mandalas. Each one told a story of connection. Once we invited friends over to help paint a pride mandala on the outside wall of my studio. We designed a bee-themed mandala for an apiarist friend and spent a week painting it with him on a building overlooking his ranch. When the mural was done, my new partner and I decided to move out of Los Angeles and into this little town that we'd inaugurated with Hope's art.

After that, Hope painted a mandala based on the St. Francis prayer and filled it with every animal we could imagine. After years of intense imagery with cuts, violence, conflict, and drama, my artwork had become a haven of peace.

I realized another paradox, one that I hadn't been strong enough to experience before. *I become stronger by being more vulnerable.*

Sharing myself with others drew them into my inner circle. When I communicated my deepest fears with my partner after an argument, instead of defending my position, the resentments disappeared, and we became closer. Facing the innocent, raw, vulnerable inner child gave me more power than I'd ever known.

I was no longer alone—inside or out.

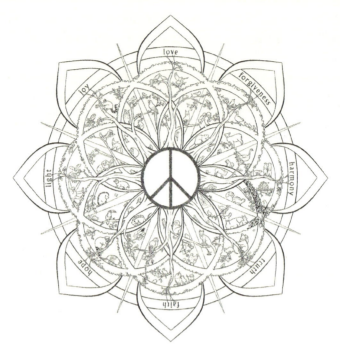

Figure 10: Line drawing for the painting titled "St. Francis Prayer/11th Step Mandala," 2012.

Your Experience

The poet Mary Oliver was one of the best at describing what is difficult to put into words. She created something akin to the beauty she was trying to capture. She, too, suffered from a rough childhood in Ohio—and turned to poetry for salvation. She found creative inspiration in the natural world around her. Her verses ache with the beauty of impermanence and the impermanence of beauty.

What inspires your creativity? Music, poetry, books, TV shows? Manga, Dungeons & Dragons, video games? Your children or pets?

Take a moment to acknowledge those teachers and how they've shaped your life.

What Hope and I can share with you is this—after pain and darkness comes light. It happens naturally, but we can also urge it along. The joy of creating is sometimes enough in itself. But other times, we need to focus on positive rituals to uplift the practice.

The purpose of these exercises is to help you connect with your littlest part—the innocent one who loved life before it got hard. No matter how cynical you might be now, you can drop in and connect with that feeling. You were once that person—they haven't gone away. So, open your heart and mind, and follow me in.

Grounding Technique: Mindful Observing

Pick an object within arm's reach—a flower, a leaf, a piece of food, a purse, a lamp—and start to notice its details. Describe what it looks like—its color, size, texture, shape, etc. Reach out and touch it. What does it feel like in your hand? Is it cold, warm, scratchy, gooey, rough, or soft? Does it make a sound when you hold it to your ear? What does it smell like? Taste like? Narrate it in as descriptive words as possible.

Stay with that one thing, looking for more that you hadn't seen before.

Now hold it against your heart. Say to yourself, *This object is real. I am real. I am part of the world around me.*

Let it go with gratitude. Sense your presence within your five senses. Note what you hear, see, smell, taste, and feel against your skin. Inhabit your self.

Exercise: A Forest Bath

In Japan, the term *Shinrin-yoku*, or "forest bathing," was coined in 1982 to describe the therapeutic effects of spending time among trees. It's not the first example of humanity turning to the woods for healing but is certainly one of the more salient in today's world. South Koreans officially promote forest therapy, as do Finns. It's becoming a new trend in California.

Numerous studies have documented the positive effects of forest bathing on the immune system, mental health, and stress levels. But it isn't just walking among trees that produces these benefits. It's the mindfulness part of the exercise that brings it home. And that's been my experience, as Hope showed me how to connect with the natural world.

Being half-Finnish, I know about feeling connected to Nature. I resisted it for many years, as I lived in Los Angeles and valued the culture of the city, but when my partner and I moved to Northern California, I visited my first redwood forest. It reminded me of childhood explorations in the nature preserve near our house in Ohio, and exploring the woods of Michigan's Upper Peninsula and Montana with my cousins. Inside a temple of trees, the air is richer. Sounds slow down. The light dims, the eyes adjust. Every ray of sun, every rustle, is part of a larger surrounding body. If you stop in the middle of it, you can feel its soul.

Bringing our creativity into the woods gives us an opportunity to commune with this soul. Find a forest or park near you. Bring your journal and pen along. Walk through slowly, taking time to notice the sounds, smells, and sights in a new way. Take deep breaths. Feel the oxygen-rich air filling your lungs. Listen with your heart.

Find the tree that speaks to you the most deeply. Sit with it. Invite it to share what it's seen over its long life.

Consider how a tree forms. If grown in isolation with no influencing factors, it would grow by the law of fractals—one branch splitting into two smaller versions of itself, then those branches would do the same, then again in perfect order, and again, *ad infinitum*. It would end up perfectly symmetrical, each pattern of branches mimicking the last as it got progressively smaller into infinity.

But trees don't grow in isolation. They're harassed by the wind, soaked by storms, burned by lightning, chewed by bugs, and sickened by disease. Branches break off, which disturbs the initial growth pattern. Birds build nests and poke holes. The bark gnarls and thickens into a story that spans longer lifetimes than ours.

Ask yourself, as you run your fingers over its skin, *What has it seen? What has it lost? Where are its wounds?* What story of comfort and wisdom would the tree share with you, if you could understand its language?

The roots extend beneath the ground, far beyond sight, drawing nourishment from the soil, communicating with fungi mycelium—sort of like a central nervous system for the entire forest. Lichen joins this symbiosis, combining fungus and algae or bacteria to form a substance that covers approximately six percent of the earth's surface. Trees of different species communicate with each other via chemical messages through this vast web of interconnected matter in a conversation of mutual help. Those with more resources share their nutrition with the ones in need. News of impending disease travels across miles, allowing others to prepare a defense. "Mother" trees are larger hubs that nurture the seedlings in the understory. Redwoods grow their "babies" in a ring around them, feeding them with their own root systems, then when they eventually die off and return to the soil, they continue to nourish their offspring.

Listen to the larger family around you. What are they saying to each other? Do they notice you? What does a non-human consciousness feel like? What would it say about you? Don't mix it up with your ego-based thoughts or habitual criticism. Listen for what it's really saying about you, to you, for you.

Now, draw that tree. It might be a literal representation of the exterior, or an imagined map of its root system. Perhaps it's a mother holding some ancient sorrow. Maybe it's reaching toward the sun. Control your pen only enough to keep it on the page—let the tree do the talking here. Tell its story in images.

When you're done, thank it. Take a moment to appreciate what you drew, and to celebrate your willingness and openness. Breathe in the mystery.

You can do this exercise in any environment or for any natural object that brings you peace. Water itself could be your guide. Be open to communicating with it, and let it speak to the innocent one inside of you, the one who still remembers that ancient language echoing inside us.

Exercise: Coloring Mandalas

A *mandala* (Sanskrit for "circle") is a circular pattern that carries meaning and function in different cultures around the world. It first appeared in Hindu texts about 3,000 years ago, but it was probably used long before then. For centuries, religious and philosophical cultures throughout Asia, Europe, the Middle East, and the Americas have used circular geometry to map and connect with spiritual hierarchies and to make sense of their place in the natural world. Tibetans often use them to build up a mental image that generates insights and achieves balance between the self and spirit. Navajo sand-painting traditions invoke Holy People to guide aspirants into their true state of Beauty and communion with the cosmos. Celtic knots and spirals featured interlacing lines with no end, and were drawn to connect to ancestors, visualize goals, stimulate spiritual growth, symbolize values, and represent the endless cycles of life.

This exercise requires a set of colored pencils. The activity of coloring lowers stress and organizes the mind. Focusing on a mandala can bring in a more spiritual energy.

We'll be creating our own mandalas in the next chapter, but for now, we're just coloring for fun. You can download free mandala templates drawn by Hope from www.stoppingselfharm.com, or you can purchase one of the many mandala-related coloring books out there.

Instead of coloring in front of the television, make this a more intentional exercise. Light a candle, play some music, ask your little one inside to come out and play. Notice which hues you like best, appreciate the sound of the pencil scratching across paper. If you feel an urge to color outside the lines, or create your own shape within the larger one, go ahead. Let the activity become a meditation with your inner child. Kids often dislike being questioned directly—so this is a way of easing in by asking them questions as they play. Approach each shape with a sense of curiosity.

Afterward, write about any thoughts or insights that came up. If you didn't have any, write about how it felt to relax into the work. Note if you're still feeling any resistance to this experience. If you are, honor it—there is no wrong way to do this.

Exercise: Bugs to Butterflies

Another symbol that is rich with meaning, color, and metaphor is the butterfly. There's a story about a child who heard something struggling inside a cocoon, so she cracked it open. A butterfly emerged—but it sank to the ground, too weak to fly. Because the kid had freed it too soon, it hadn't struggled long enough to build up wing strength. The metaphor for us is that we each need our suffering to hone the skills we need to emerge in a new form.

Why don't you try doing some research on butterflies? We all know what Monarchs look like, but what about the Mourning Cloak, the Admiral, the Tortoiseshell, or the Red-Bodied Swallowtail? Do some drawings of their colorful patterns. Teach yourself how to draw a wing outline. Learn how many segments are in a butterfly body. Once you learn how they're structured and why, it's easier to draw one, even if you don't consider yourself an artist. Remember when you filled out the stick figure with a body and a round head? It's the same with any creature—round-ish head, tube for the body, and appendages (legs, wings, antennae, etc.).

Another option is to do some free-association writing about butterflies. Think of all the words inspired by them—caterpillar, cocoon, metamorphosis, chrysalis, flutter, flower. Create some sentences using these words in a different context. *I was cocooned for so long that when I finally completed my metamorphosis, my wings were strong as steel.*

Your little one might prefer a different creature. Hope is obsessed with ladybugs. That's how I found out that each of the common red and black varieties has exactly seven spots. I've drawn my share of ladybugs, caterpillars, and snails. What are your favorites?

Remember how fascinating everything seemed when you were a kid? It's because everything was brand new—and infused with magic and life. I used to think everything had its own feelings, even rocks. I'd go into the garden or the woods and have deep conversations with the natural world. Today, I tune into that same observing power to connect with Spirit in Nature. Sometimes, I talk to my roses. I listen for wisdom from trees.

I bet that if you set aside judgment and look around through the eyes of your innocent child, you'll see the magic that's still there.

Exercise: Creative Kids

If you still don't consider yourself an artist, this exercise might change your mind. Children don't worry about how their art looks; they just love to create.

So, find a real kid to draw with.

On a blank piece of paper, ask them to draw a line. Any shape, any style. Then use that squiggle as a starting point—and create an object around it. Make a curved line into a whale, or a ghost—whatever is easiest. Then *you* draw a line and challenge them to create something from it. Switch roles again.

Once they get started, they won't want to stop.

Let your inner kid play with them. Ask questions. Let them tell stories. Drawing is not just a primal instinct, it's a fundamental human right—and co-creating with another little one is the best way to remind ourselves of that.

While we're emulating children and their ease with creativity, let's extend that to other activities. What about taking a gentle yoga or stretching class—with the intention of playing rather than working out? Same with dancing or spontaneous movement. No one can see you cut loose in your own bedroom. Or you could try something more tactile like a pottery class—throw pots, sculpt clay, get your hands dirty. Go to a sound bath class at a yoga center, find a drumming circle, join a choir, or jam session. Find ways to play and create that work best for you and where you live.

Advanced Exercise: Mindful Creating

Take whatever insect or animal you focused on in the butterflies exercise and develop it into a series within your favorite medium. But don't just document them—ask what they mean to you, and what they express in your art.

Here's an example. Once when my partner and I were trimming a small tree at our house, we found an empty hummingbird nest on the ground. We'd accidentally knocked it loose. A little more searching revealed a tiny baby bird. It was still alive.

We placed it carefully back in the nest and put it back into what was left of the branches. We went inside and watched from the window to see if its mother would return. Much to my relief, she finally did. Over the next two weeks, that mom continued to feed its baby. It was the rainy season, so I rigged an umbrella over the branch to protect it from the storms. It slowly grew, and its spiky fuzz turned into feathers.

But one day, I found its lifeless body just outside the nest, its neck broken by some predator. I was heartbroken. I cried more about that baby bird than I had since Shilo passed. The only thing that brought me comfort was painting its portrait. That sparked a whole series of tiny hummingbird paintings, each of them in a dynamic background, shouting out some protest. To me, they symbolized the fragile power of small things and the desire to be seen and protected.

Artists throughout the centuries have turned to the natural world for inspiration. My mother paints and sculpts all kinds of spirit animals. Birds symbolize her voice, bears are sacred protectors, and owls carry wisdom. These animals weave through her work and tell stories through their eyes.

Find a little spirit animal of your own and paint them in different poses and environments. Research the different varieties and species. What do they embody in your psyche? How do you feel toward them? Do you want to do small, intimate portraits or large epics? Follow where they lead you.

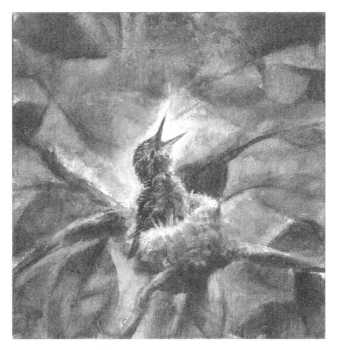

Figure 11: "Don't Go!" Oil on 6" x 6" board, 2019.

Visualization: Bring it Home

This time, we're doing the visualization at the end of this chapter's exercises, not at the beginning. That's because little kids who've had their trust violated need time to relax and come out from hiding.

The easiest way to coax them out is to engage them in play. Once we've done that, they'll be more open with us.

As usual, find a comfortable place to sit. Cover yourself with a warm, soothing blanket. Let go of your preconceived notions and judgment. Approach this exercise with an open mind.

Close your eyes and breathe into and out of your heart.

Search inside your body for that part that enjoyed coloring, connecting with the tree, and dancing. Feel him/her/them moving around inside you. Wrap your arms around yourself, smile, and thank that part of you for coming out to play. Send love through your arms to envelop that energy. Feel their gratitude and trust. Note any sensations beneath your skin.

Ask that part of you, *Do you have a name? Where do you live?* Let them take your hand and show you around their world. Share in their delight. Treat them as you would your child or pet. Feel how they receive your adoration.

This time, activate the adult part of you a little more than you have thus far. Envision holding them in your lap. You might rock a little. Ask them how it feels when the self-harming part takes over. Talk to them gently about how you're working with that part to learn new behaviors. It's like you're comforting your youngest child who has been hurt by an older sibling. You're learning new parenting skills, so this is awkward and you're afraid you'll mess up, but the little one knows you love them, and you know it, too. Admit that you're not perfect, and that you'll continue to make mistakes. The family is learning new ways of communicating.

But unlike a parent out in the world, you are both the adult *and* the little one—so you can ask them to help you with the part that self-harms. Ask them to bring their superpowers of innocence, love, and play. Maybe the next time the desire to hurt comes up, that little part can enact some mischief to make everyone laugh.

Assure them that you are open to hearing messages anytime, and you'll do your best to meet any needs as they come up.

When you're ready to come out of the meditation, take some deep breaths, ground your body, and open your eyes. Again, write about what you experienced. Share it. Celebrate your progress.

If you've connected with the part that self-harms and the innocent child inside, you've done amazing work already. Most people never get this far. All these aspects of yourself belong to you, and no one else.

Reflection and Concluding Thoughts

Rather than writing about this process, let yourself feel it. Notice the world around you, take it in. Do you feel any different now than you did when you started this book? Do you have more hope?

As I said, this book is not about making a vow of abstinence. The resolve to stop has to come from inside, not from external forces. The part of us that wants to self-harm is a *silencer*—it doesn't want the innocent one to have needs, to be in pain, or to express itself, because that's dangerous. It leads to rejection or abuse. We were taught that behavior from caregivers who didn't know any other way.

It's time now to do things differently, to *listen* to what our child voices are trying to say. It's time to listen to our wounds and allow the long-buried innocence to re-emerge.

When we access parts of us that have been stuck, frozen, or imprisoned, we release energy. Think of a glacier melting—it raises water levels around the world. The same is true of our own psyches. Long-buried parts of us wake and stretch, eager to live again. It can feel invigorating. It can also be scary, and it's common to retreat into familiar habits. Change is hard—which is why most of us prefer to stay the same, even if it hurts.

We still have more to do, but it gets easier as time goes on. Things start making more sense. We can feel the change in the air. Puzzle pieces are falling into place as we begin understanding ourselves and trusting in the journey.

The next chapter will provide tools to keep the momentum going.

"There is a place in the soul that neither time nor space nor no created thing can touch."

—Meister Eckhart

"In order to work and to become an artist one needs love. At least, one who wants sentiment in his work must in the first place feel it himself, and live with his heart."

—Vincent Van Gogh

CHAPTER SEVEN

LOVE THE WORK

The long slog of healing requires discipline and sustained practice. A ship doesn't turn on a dime—it eases slowly toward its new path. It's the same with us. Breaking through old blocks might make us think we're done, we're through to the other side, we're all good now. Then with the first setback, we despair. Perhaps that breakthrough wasn't real after all. We always knew this wouldn't work. It's easier to reach for the tried-and-true self-harming than to test out new behaviors, especially in the midst of being overwhelmed.

That's why it's important to have a daily routine to deepen our new grooves of habit. As Steve Chandler said, "The human spirit, like a campfire, must be lit again each day."[17] No one is immune from having to re-light their own fire.

An old axiom states that discipline equals happiness. And I've found this to be true. One of the first things people learn in recovery programs is to make their bed every morning. It's surprising how that one small thing makes such a difference. During the worst of

---

[17] Steve Chandler, *Re-Inventing Yourself, Revised Edition: How to Become the Person You've Always Wanted to Be* (Red Wheel, Revised Edition, 2005), 204.

their "bottom," addicts can barely function—so reassembling the bed brings them back into normal living. Another routine is to pray and meditate at a regular time each day, preferably upon awakening. Not only does that set the day off right, but it also establishes and feeds a connection with self and with God/Spirit. Any relationship needs time and investment to flourish—and our relationship with the deepest part of ourselves is the most valuable one of all. It's vital to put in the time to keep that healthy.

To people who have self-harmed, the concept of self-control is foreign or even unsafe. I used to associate the word "discipline" with "punishment." The connection to my father's abuse seems obvious now, but it took me many years to see it. I prided myself on my discipline—I exercised, ate well, worked hard, stayed sober, read books, and accomplished things. But I was always aware that my rigid rules were vulnerable to upheaval at any moment. And the underlying motivation was still harmful. I exercised and ate well to control my figure (which I hated anyway), I worked hard to make money (that I knew would leak away), I read books to search for answers to my despair (without doing what those books recommended). I prayed to Spirit for relief, for security, for happiness. But I never asked how I could be of service to Spirit.

Amor fati is Latin for "love of one's fate." By dwelling in my suffering, I was resisting my fate—resisting my suffering—my life as it *is* on a daily basis. It wasn't on purpose—I could no more escape my morass of thoughts than I could leap to the moon. I tried every path, every labyrinth, every loophole, but I always ended up right where I began, with the same old thoughts and fears.

But there is another way—not an escape, or an upheaval, but a gentle easing in. Note that *amor fati* begins with the word *love*. That is the secret key. We don't get to acceptance without love.

Otherwise, it's just resignation. Love turns out to be the greatest partner, the greatest tool.

When we use love as the lens through which we experience life, everything changes.

Here's one example of how I apply love to my daily behaviors. I ask myself now, before I exercise: Is this out of love or hate? Am I forcing myself to swim outdoors in the pouring rain because it feels good afterward, or because that voice is telling me I'm fat? Am I really up to it today? Am I putting this food into my mouth to nourish my body, or to escape my feelings, and prove once more that I'm out of control? Am I staying up late to read that book because it's changing my life for the better, or because I don't care about being sleep-deprived?

Another way to use this shift in perspective is to love my fate—which to me means loving everything that happened to me. This is not the same as letting other people off the hook. It means I accept what I cannot change and love who I've become as a result. I love Faith for enduring the abuse and finding creative ways to survive and thrive, and Hope for going to sleep so she could preserve her innocence. I love my imperfections—they're what make me human and connect me to other imperfect people. I love the traffic because I'm lucky enough to have a car (and don't have to ride the bus like I did in my early twenties). I love my work because it builds skills, earns money, keeps me busy, and gives me a purpose. I love the storm because it's so beautiful afterward when the sun comes out. I love the setback because it gives me an opportunity to try something else. This is not denial. It's more of a recalibration. I still feel anger and work to change things I'm passionate about, but I can choose how I respond to events, rather than being ruled by emotion.

Love is also an organizing force. Being inside a fragmented mind makes it very hard to practice discipline. But with love as our guide, we can begin to structure our thoughts—and subsequently, our lives—with more agency and confidence.

We may not have learned this growing up, if our caregivers used the word in the context of abuse or neglect—but love, in its truest sense, is trustworthy. It persists. We can have faith in love; it gives us hope.

Love is what connects us to the world. I used to yearn for enough love to come in and fill that hole inside me—but I never received enough from others, no matter how hard I tried to gain their approval. But when I am of service to another person, love flows through me and fills me up. I have to trust that as it passes through and outward, more will always return if I continue to give it away. I let go and have faith.

Many say that God is Love. Whether we call it God, Creator, Universe, Nature, Great Spirit, Lady of Light, Creative Intelligence, the Mystery, whatever—it's an essential energy underlying all of life.

When I cut myself, the wounds healed. I didn't suture tissue back together from the bottom up—an intelligent process did that all on its own. It's the same with healing our psyches. There's an innate pull toward health inside each of us. It's creative, life-giving, and always evolving. The fastest way to tap into it is by giving love.

Love is also what initiates us into a greater purpose in life, which is to transform not only our suffering, but that of others. As the psychologist and Jung's colleague Marie-Louise von Franz said in *The Problem of the Puer Aeternus*:

> One has to be wounded in order to become a healer. This is the local image of a universal mythological motif, which is described in Eliade's book about the initiation of medicine men and shamans. Nobody becomes either one or the other without

first having been wounded, either cut open by the initiator and having certain magical stones inserted into his body, or a spear thrown at his neck, or some such thing. Generally, the experiences are ecstatic—stars or ghost-like demons hit them or cut them open—but always they have to be pierced or cut apart before they become healers, for that is how they acquire the capacity for healing others.[18]

And so, once again, we must go within to reclaim this legacy.

My Experience

The third internal part rose to the surface gradually. I'd always known she was there. She was the pre-teen who became a teenager and then aged along with me. But she wasn't *me*—the consciousness who lived in my adult life—she was the shadowy underbelly, the one who carried unwanted feelings like shame, terror, and hatred.

The "I" that looked back from the mirror, the 40-something woman who entered her second big cycle of therapy in life, was still detached from the teenager inside. She still felt like a deadened husk that I dragged along and tried to ignore.

Once I connected with her, she told me her name was "L." At first, I thought she said, "Elle," but she clarified that it's the *letter* L. She didn't tell me what it stood for.

I didn't want to spend time with her at first. It felt super uncomfortable. My adult self-assurance evaporated, and I was that awkward pre-pubescent girl again. My clothes felt too tight, fears dammed up in my throat. Whenever L came around, I believed

---

[18] Maria-Louise Von Franz, *The Problem of the Puer Aeturnus* (Inner City Books, 3rd Edition, 2000), 116.

that no one liked me, even my therapist. Every anxiety turned into a catastrophe. She woke me up at three a.m. to obsess about every mistake. Her voice hounded me with doomsday predictions. *Everyone you love will die or leave. You're going to run out of money and end up homeless. You're fooling yourself that you're a good artist because you're just a dilettante.* Dilettante? Really? I have no idea where she found that old-fashioned word, but it hounded me for years.

It was easy to trace those words back to my parents. I'd internalized their anxieties and projections, like every kid does. But L had sharpened them into vitriolic punches that tormented me day in and day out. As a young person, L had tried to make sense of everything, using her limited tools and broken role models. The adult Maggie could reason her way out of dilemmas, but L had no use for rationality. In her world, powerful forces could descend at any time and obliterate her security. She had only a tiny lighter inside a vast, dark cave. No amount of reasoning could convince her that things were okay.

When I finally turned back to listen to what she was trying to tell me, I plunged deeper into her world. She reminded me what it was like to be that age. And she told me her story.

L was "born" when I was eleven and living in London with my family—our second European visit. My father had been given a sabbatical grant to study theaters and the arts. Two of my uncles were living there with their families, so we often visited them. It sounds like a wonderful time, and in many ways, it was, except that my parents were preoccupied with their struggles, and I was often left alone. I figured out the subway system and traveled from one end of the city to another. Once I was supposed to meet my mother after school at one uncle's flat, only to find out when I arrived that she'd told me the wrong uncle's address, and I had to find my way across town to the other one.

Because we lived on a tight budget, we rented a sparse, poorly heated flat from an artist in a gritty part of the city. Every room held some strange piece of art. One was empty except for a hole in the wall that gave a small glimpse of the other room, which contained only a column topped with a pile of stones. Dad insisted it was haunted by an old Scottish ghost who sang whenever I practiced my violin—yet another reason to fear the world around me. The girls' school I attended held a scary tableau of poverty, smoking, fighting, and rage. I adapted well on the outside, but secretly, I grappled with terror every day. After we returned to Ohio, I brought those ghosts home with me.

The next year, at age twelve, L's first full year at the co-ed middle school in the next town over, she lost all ability to make friends. Suddenly, she was an outcast. Her loneliness stretched to the edges of her world and beyond. When Faith's surges took over, she's the one who learned to numb the skin. She self-poisoned with pills; she slept fifteen hours a night to escape consciousness. She ate to try and fill the hole inside, and when she hated her bulging stomach and hips in the mirror, she stuck her finger down her throat to purge her insides.

She yearned for affection from her alcoholic father and distant mother, and believed she was unlovable at her core. While her father steered the car and drank vodka from a 7 Up can, L watched the dividing line on the road, convinced that if she took her eyes off it, the car would crash. She sat vigil while he nodded off on the couch and waited for the lit cigar to fall from his hand so she could pick it up and stop the whole house from burning down. She thought she had to stay alert to keep the world from ending; yet at the same time, she felt paralyzed by depression. Despite her vow never to drink like her dad, L took up drinking at fourteen as a way to connect with him.

She's also the one who dealt with confusing feelings about girls. Being LGBTQ+ was far from cool in the early 1980s. So, she kept her feelings secret and, instead, became promiscuous with boys. From age fifteen on, every time she drank, she ended up doing things that were shameful, embarrassing, confusing, and sometimes dangerous. The line of consent was crossed more than once, but the word "no" only came out in a whisper.

L was the one who attempted suicide at seventeen. That alerted other adults that she needed help. Although she wasn't able to share much from her inner world, she found a savior in Mrs. Hren, and a lifeline to a hopeful future.

At the same time, L was responsible for many of the gifts that helped the whole system survive. She's the one who used her brain to figure things out, who played Dungeons & Dragons and created new worlds. She loved puzzles, games, and riddles. She liked to reason out problems until a solution could be carved away from the noise. A hatred of the adolescent body led to a fierce dedication to competitive swimming, which taught self-esteem and discipline.

Her hard work led to a full scholarship to college, a way out of Ohio, and a ticket to California where she knew she'd find other gay people. And indeed, she did. L is the one who, despite her loneliness and fear, found the courage to come out and join the growing ranks of young queer people in Los Angeles. Her interest in worldbuilding led to a career designing theme parks. She got to create castles, carousels, cartoon-shaped stores, dragon-themed roller coasters, hedge mazes with talking unicorns and gargoyles, and so much more.

As Maggie matured into the adult woman that people saw on the outside, L grew as well. Not as quickly, but steadily, in her own way. Part of that awkward pre-teen stayed stuck at twelve years old, but part of her evolved as the fragmented adult made her way into middle age.

I was finally able to appreciate L's gifts. I could see and *feel* her strength, her shy sweetness. In fact, I began to see *all* the gifts that came from my parts and how they'd managed the aftereffects of trauma. I realized that Faith is my strength, my voice, and my inner warrior. He steers me away from dangerous situations. Hope is the magical one—she brings play and laughter, and delights in the natural world. And L can solve any problem that comes my way. She's also good at helping others solve their problems.

I realized there are flip sides to our trauma responses—and they can become our greatest strengths. Because I know how to dissociate, I can easily let go of bodily stress during meditation. Years of anxious thinking trained my brain to sift quickly through stimuli to find clarity at the heart of chaos. A lifetime of hypervigilance has made me extra observant. Being overly sensitive has taught me to be gentle with myself and others. Surviving great pain gave me compassion for others. And not being able to trust reality made it easier for me to accept the possibility of a Spirit realm beyond the reach of my intellect. In fact, it helped me experience it on a visceral level that I might not have without the jarring traumas that knocked me out of a comfortable existence.

It turns out that L, the one who is most solitary, doesn't actually *like* to be alone. She thrives most when she's connected to Faith and Hope as a family. Then, she's able to trust enough to share herself with others. She wants to be able to let go of the wheel. She—and we—can't do this alone. She was my key to being able to connect authentically with others.

Maybe you've guessed what L stands for, but it took me a surprisingly long time. Maybe that's because she's secretive and didn't want to reveal it. When I finally asked for her real name, she rolled her eyes and said, *Duh. It's Love.*

And so, L taught me about love. As David Hawkins states in his book, *Letting Go*, "[Love] is more than an emotion or a thought—it is a state of being. Love is what we have become through the pathway of surrender."[19]

That's true of everything, really. The things we hold onto the tightest are destined to leave us. Goal setting and striving are useful, but only up to a point. The rest is up to fate, or chance, or God. If we don't love the work itself, we'll always be miserable.

I used to think I was doing the work to reach my predetermined destination—but as it turns out, the work *is* the reward. It's what gives us the gifts we desire.

Paradox number six—*the journey is the destination*.

There is no wizard behind the curtain. There is only growth, evolution, becoming. On a spiritual path, we are always at the beginning. It's circular, not linear—we are cycling deeper into ourselves, not going somewhere else.

Belief in a higher power is also a process. It's constantly evolving, being challenged, emerging into new forms. The search for God *is* God. The point of prayer is not to get something—the point of prayer (in all its forms) is to be with Spirit.

Once when I was painting murals in a theme park just outside Tokyo, a friend and I took the train to Kamakura, a city of temples, known for its giant Buddha statue. We memorized the Japanese characters for the Great Buddha and set out on the trail closest to the train station. At every fork in the road, we followed the signs with the correct letters. Along the way, we passed through small temples and shrines. At one, statues of foxes filled the grounds,

---

[19] David Hawkins, *Letting Go: The Pathway of Surrender* (Hay House, 2013, Kindle Edition), 172.

and squirrels ran up our arms to get treats. At another, we washed our money in a cave. But after a couple of hours with no food, we started wondering where in the heck this Buddha statue might be. Hunger gnawed at us.

We found an English-speaking hiker, who explained to us that we were on the Great Buddha *trail*, not the pathway to the statue! So, we slid down the mountainside through heavy brush back to the road and within minutes, we finally entered the grounds of the Great Buddha. He towered over forty feet above us, looking serenely down. All those hours of hiking and he was just around the corner the whole time. But if we hadn't gone on that adventure, we'd never have seen all those amazing temples.

I'll never forget the sense of peace that washed over me as I realized, with some amusement, that it wasn't the destination that mattered—walking the Great Buddha trail of life was the whole point.

Your Experience

Healing isn't a destination—it's a discipline. Even after breakthroughs have been achieved and corners turned, there's always more work to do.

But each awakening releases more joy for the work itself. It's like walking through a jail and unlocking cells so that prisoners can come out and join your army. Each time one emerges, they shed their past and enter the sunlight of the spirit with you. It's constant upward progress. Even if it's three steps forward and two steps back, we still gain a step.

Creativity doesn't just help the process; it *is* the process. Each journey is unique and requires faith in our imagination and our ability to forge a new path. Perhaps instead of calling it a "long slog," I might use the term "grand puzzle." Every life has a puzzle of its own to solve—which leads to the gift that we are meant to offer the world.

L taught me that love and creativity aren't just about expressing something—they're a way to organize the chaos, suture wounds, and connect with others. Her specialty is unraveling knots.

Once those strands are free, they can be put to good use.

This chapter has a lot of exercises because L loves to solve puzzles. Each exercise becomes a foundation for further exploration, fueled by imagination and willingness. I've used all of these activities myself and have slowly transformed old habits into productive new superpowers.

Grounding Technique: Three A.M. Lists

Most of us know that dreaded awakeness at ungodly hours of the morning. It's usually a bad dream that wakes me up—some fevered experience of rejection, or disaster, or frustration, or battle. The more my thoughts try to solve problems, the bigger they loom.

For me, that's the time when L spins into anxiety. Admonishing her to go back to sleep does nothing. Praying doesn't help, either. The only tool that seems to work is a gratitude list.

The benefits of gratitude lists have been established through empirical studies. Anyone who has tried this practice for any length of time knows how helpful it can be. I've done it for years, and it's slowly turned my pessimism into optimism. It gave me new glasses to view the world.

But mostly, it's soothing. The brain needs something to occupy it until sleep takes over the body. Just counting sheep isn't enough—that's boring and random. L needs a sense of purpose to keep her going.

So, I list my gratitudes alphabetically. I think of as many things I appreciate that start with the letter A. Or I'll pick one thing for each letter and go through to Z (I can't tell you how many times I've expressed gratitude for xylophones and zebras!). I take time to appreciate each thing and fill my heart with love for it. That way, it not only focuses my thoughts, but it also fills my body with peace. It bothers me less that my mind is perseverating if I'm training it on positive things.

Try this the next time you're caught in an insomnia whirlpool. Instead of trying to shut the brain down, give it a happy task. Thank that part of you for being so vigilant. Appeal to their strengths to ease you back into sleep.

Visualization: The Great Buddha Trail

Remember in chapter four when you descended into your ideal environment to meet your spirit guide? We're going to re-visit that place—but with a new lens.

Sit in a comfortable place and close your eyes. Take three deep, gentle breaths through your nose. Scan your body for any knots or numb spots. Breathe into them, let go of resistance. Picture your teenager from the inside—what it felt like to be that age. Where in your body do they live? Does your physical awareness change as you embody that age? Send loving energy into that sensation. Let go some more.

Feel yourself dropping downward. You can recall the elevator exercise, or you can simply sink to the bottom on your own. Breathe out any last traces of tightness. Surrender it all.

Settle into that environment you've chosen as your happy place—forest, beach, water, mountains, desert, whatever. Enter this space with curiosity and anticipation. You're embarking on a pathway of discovery, and you can feel the experience calling you forward. You can also sense your spirit guide or God energy waiting at the end, always there, in no hurry at all.

This time, notice details more. As you begin to walk, notice if you're alone or if any of your inner parts are with you. Are you in an adult body or a child's? What are you wearing? What's on your feet? Notice the sensation against your skin. Are you stepping over roots, sinking into sand, or swimming in water? What does the air feel like?

Perhaps you come upon that tree you met in the woods in chapter six. Here, in the realm of Spirit, its energy is crystal clear. It greets you with a familiar wave of love. You lean against it, feel its heart beating, and listen to the wind rustle through its leaves. What does the bark smell like? Are there birds or animals around? Sense the magic in this environment. Let it resonate with your littlest one inside. Let them show you around. Feel the endless wonderment, notice small things.

Listen to the impulse calling you forward. It sparks some excitement in your belly. You carry that littlest one with you along as you follow that summons. The path unfolds before you. What do you see and hear? Are there any critters with you? How does the light move?

Soon, you come upon the one who used to cut—but they're not big and scary, they're small and dear. You scoop them into your arms. Their gratitude washes over you and connects with a click inside your heart. What is that being saying to you? What do they look like? Where are you in the environment—is there any special landmark that marks this spot where you met? How does this one interact with the littlest one? What are they feeling inside your body? What do they point out for you to notice?

The energy is still calling you forward—so you continue onward with your little ones. How does the environment change as you venture deeper? Is there a scent? Is there music? Do you hear water, birds, or wind?

Finally, you come upon the core Spirit of this place. It's been waiting for you all along, here at your Source. Your teenager is there, smiling at you, happy to see you finally made it here. The Spirit opens up and all of you settle inside. From here, you look out on the world with peace. Nothing is solid. Everything is moving energy, lit from within. Feel the Oneness all around and your body within it. See how you've created the images and sensations from the textures of your own life experience—and see how they're only shimmering skins on the reality beneath. Both the surface and the underlying shape are real. One is the wave; one is deep water—but both are the ocean. Accept it all.

When you feel ready, surface gently. Put both hands over your heart. Thank your inner ones, the experience, and yourself for being willing. Open your eyes. Return to your day but with your new awareness still cradled inside.

Exercise: Gratitude

We're returning to the healing power of gratitude lists but in a more tactile way.

I once did a self-portrait where I wrote everything I was grateful for on the arms and chest. The overall image was meant to portray the experience of transcendence through acknowledging all the people and spiritual practices that had gotten me there. That was before I relapsed in cutting and worked to find healing, but it was still a powerful exercise. It grounded me and affirmed I had a bigger Self beyond my body.

So, let's try a version of that here. Either in your journal or on a bigger sheet of paper, draw a figure representing you. It doesn't have to look like you. It just needs to be in the general shape of your body.

Now, start writing or drawing into that body all the things you're grateful for—everything that got you to this place, everyone you love, all the good things in your life. Even the self-harming. See it as a gift. Let your instinct guide your choices in where you place each item. Perhaps some things will be grouped together on one side of your body, some on the other. Which things dwell inside your stomach? Your heart? Anything in your toes? Write and draw until you feel complete.

A more daring version of this is to use our own skin as the canvas—similar to the one we did with the red pen, but with a different angle. Gather non-toxic, skin-safe felt tip pens (or even makeup pencils) in whatever colors you like. Take off your clothes and look at your reflection in the mirror. Summon your teenage self. You may feel awkward, stupid, resentful, embarrassed, or angry. Maybe you'll feel inspired. Don't fight it—just observe with compassion. This is the skin that has grown with you, that has endured wounds, that absorbs input, that provides a membrane between you and the world. See if you can let go of judgment.

When you're ready, write something you're grateful for somewhere on your body. Take the time to ask your interior parts what to write next and where. Treat it as a sacred exercise of tattooing. You're telling your story on the temple of you. Write whatever comes up, but steer it into positive words and statements. Draw pictures if you want. Let this be an embodiment of gratitude.

Before you wash it all off, take a picture of your tattooed self. Today you're an art piece.

Sometimes it takes me years to discover what a painting was trying to say. The same may be true of this painting of you. Whatever our creative voice expresses holds some wisdom for us. When we're ready to hear it, it will feel obvious.

Exercise: Putting the Pieces Back Together

Kintsugi, a Japanese term translated as "golden joinery," is the traditional art of repairing broken pottery using gold or silver lacquer. It's a process of honoring the object's history by highlighting its cracks. It also reflects a wider philosophy—by showcasing the imperfect "wounds" in a piece, one meditates on non-attachment, the inevitability of change, and identification with things outside of the self.

It's easy to see why this concept is a rich source of inspiration for many modern artists and culture makers. The practice of mending broken parts isn't limited to ceramics and gold paste.

Clothing designers, jewelers, collage artists, sculptors, painters, and more have utilized it in their work to explore metaphors of imperfection and repair. My own work echoes these themes—but I paint the "cracks" or wounds first, then build up paint around that, assembling fragmented shapes into a whole with the scars forming the seams.

In this version of *kintsugi*, we're going to create a collage. We'll focus on what we're trying to repair—the damaged self.

You'll need a big piece of paper, scissors, glue, a photo or print of yourself, and whatever images you want to include from photos, magazines, or other sources.

Close your eyes, take a deep breath, and scan your body from the inside. Extend your awareness into your fingers and toes, feel your scars, note any pain or stuckness. Locate your little child and ask them to come play with you. Then open your eyes and with that inner awareness, start to cut out shapes. Assemble them roughly into a self-portrait. Include words if you want. Think about how it feels to be broken, fragmented, injured, or misunderstood. Get messy. When you like how it looks, start gluing down pieces, leaving a little space in between them. You can wait until all the pieces are cut before gluing, or you can create as you go along. The final silhouette might be square, or shaped like a person, or just random.

Once all the shards are adhered, study the piece, and ask it what it needs to fill the cracks. Red paint to simulate blood? Gold glitter? Stitches? What material can you choose that will give it coherence, strength, or joy? Enjoy the process of suturing the broken parts. Let your little kid have fun. This isn't just a collage—it's an expression of self-love.

In a way, everything we're doing in this book is *kintsugi*. We're honoring our imperfection, making it our superpower. When a broken bone heals, it's stronger in that spot than it was before the break. The scar is the gold lacquer sealing our parts back together.

Another exercise is *kintsugi*-style mask-making. You can try assembling one from scratch, but it's much easier to purchase a paintable paper mask as a base.

Gather materials that speak to your particular story. You might include instruments of self-harm, or band-aids, or perhaps photos of yourself or your wounds. I once glued dozens of X-Acto blades onto a canvas then painted a self-portrait over the top of them. I depicted myself throwing blades into the air, complete with plenty of red paint.

As you adhere pieces to the mask, tell a story of what your false self is trying to hide. Feel free to spray, cut, draw on, or otherwise alter the mask however you please. Leave space in between pieces to fill with paint, *kintsugi*-style. Whatever materials or method you choose, follow the same process as in the example above—look inward for guidance, then let yourself play. Let the creative act become an expression of healing. You're acknowledging the wound, honoring your scars, and repairing the cracks.

When you're done, put on the mask and look in the mirror. Be amazed, be proud. Tell someone what it means. In fact, put on the mask and speak from the voice that created it. Your art is your truth—and your gift. Acknowledge your courage and cleverness.

Exercise: Constructing Mandalas

In the last chapter, we called upon the littlest one to color mandalas. Now, we're going to make our own.

After learning about Tibetan mandalas during his travels, Carl Jung brought them into his therapeutic practice. He experimented with creating his own, using spontaneous shapes as they came to mind. He began to see these "cryptograms" as embodying "Formation, Transformation, Eternal Mind's eternal recreation"[20]—a path to the center, to individuation. When he directed clients to create their own cryptograms, he found that the practice often brought deep insights into their lives.

So, let's try a version of that to see what comes up. It begins with a simple circle in the middle of a page. It doesn't need to be perfect (mine never are). The point is to have fun and learn things, not stress out about imperfections. But if the thought of drawing geometric shapes makes you anxious, you can purchase a mandala-making kit online. That will help with creating basic, repeatable shapes around a circle. If you're savvy with computer design programs, you can do

---

[20] C.G. Jung, *Memories, Dreams, Reflections*, ed. Aniela Jaffé, trans. Richard and Clara Winston (Vintage Books, Revised Edition, 1989), 224.

all this digitally. Or you can download a free template from www.stoppingselfharm.com.

Start by setting a spiritual tone—light a candle, play music, meditate, say a prayer, or whatever plugs you in. You'll begin with a warm-up mandala.

Draw a circle. Divide it into sections by drawing a vertical line through the middle, then cross it horizontally so the circle is divided into four sections. Choose a simple shape to draw in one of those quadrants. Turn the paper 45 degrees and repeat that shape in the next quadrant. Don't worry if it's irregular. Do that two more times so all four pie pieces are filled.

Now, look at the shape that's emerged, and ask what it needs next. Is it calling for another piece inside a certain quadrant or a ray jumping out of the sphere? Whatever it is, duplicate it three more times as you turn the paper in a circle. Keep adding shapes as you march around the mandala. Hold your thoughts loosely as you draw, only stepping in to ask what shape comes next. Let your hands operate automatically.

You could also try one using words. Once the circle is in place, divide it into sections using words instead of lines. Let your current mood determine which ones to use. For example, if you're feeling hopeful, write words like *curious, happy, awake, timid, hope* or phrases like *trying something new, feeling a little weird, doing it anyway*. Draw them so they form the armature of the mandala. Now, write a sentence around the circle's diameter that connects those words into a story. Add new words emanating outward like rays. When you have a structure you're happy with, use colored pencils to fill the spaces in between. Choose hues that align with the words.

Let's try a mandala made of cryptograms that represent you. This time, when you draw the circle, create a shape in the center that symbolizes who you are today. Perhaps it's a face, a heart, a sun, or a peace sign. Maybe you're feeling triggered, and you want to draw a blade or a dark cloud.

Now ask that symbol, *What does it mean?* What other images does it bring to mind? A heart might call for a line of hearts stretching out to the edge of the page. If it's a dark cloud, you might draw a lightning streak outward from there. Whatever shape you draw, repeat it all the way around. With each new shape that's created, ask what's beneath that. If it's a wheel of lightning coming out of a cloud, what is it trying to tell you? Is it piercing skin, creating sparks, breaking down walls? Keep asking the cryptogram what it's trying to say until you've filled the page.

Beyond this, you can experiment with dividing the circle into more segments, creating more complex shapes, adding circles within and without, extending pieces outside, including organic shapes, coloring in collaged photographs, doing "rage art," spontaneous drawing—whatever tells a story. You might research what mandala-type geometrics were used by your ancestors. Whether your culture is European, African, Asian, Mayan, Australian, Indigenous, or mixed, there will be something in your past for you to draw upon.

Write about what you learn. Be open to the messages that come, without judgment. Creativity is a way into worlds that can't be accessed with our rational minds.

Share your mandalas with someone to see what they perceive in your work. Jung believed that this type of sacred work connected us to the collective unconscious. See what it sparks in others.

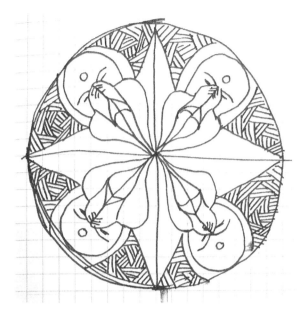

Figure 12: Example of a mandala doodle. It doesn't have to be perfect! This one taught me that I was feeling contemplative and needed to slow down to pray.

Exercise: Revise Your Map

Pull out the map you drew in chapter three (if you haven't created that yet, now is a good time). Look at it from your new place of understanding about internal parts. Is there anything you left out? Add it in now.

Can you see the milestones where fragments of you got frozen in time? What trauma stunted your growth? Mark where the parts were born. If they've given you names, write them in here. If not, just create avatars or symbols to represent them on the page. How did they survive the ensuing years? What skills did they accrue as they moved forward in time? Write those down along the path.

What spiritual help did you receive along the way? Did it come in the form of a visitation, a feeling, or a person? Name those experiences. See if they connect to a particular part. Can you trace the presence of Spirit across your life?

This is your map. It's not over yet—it's a series of chapters in an ongoing story. My friend Adele says that when we near death and look back, our lives will read like well-plotted novels. It's hard to see the end while we're in it—but we're each living a unique narrative. Whatever comes next will further develop that arc.

Hopefully, by now, you can trust that future unknown challenges can be faced, overcome, and absorbed into the story of you.

Exercise: Tracking Change

My cousin who used to cut herself from age eleven into her mid-thirties came up with ways to ground herself through documentation. She mapped her bad days in a calendar, along with the triggers. The days she cut herself were marked with a big, red X. Later, in recovery, she began to document her life through the lens of a camera. She edits all her images and videos into stories that she sends out to her mailing list. Her methods inspired this next exercise.

On a computer or by hand, draw a large grid with at least thirty squares. You could use a commercially printed calendar, but if you draw your own, it'll be easier to customize. Decide on the things you want to track—days you self-harmed or didn't, days you went to bed early, days you exercised or ate well, days you went to therapy, days you discovered something amazing. You might include the times you did an exercise from this book. It's up to you what to track. Decide on a symbol for each thing, preferably in different colors. Draw the key for each symbol on the side (or, if you want more privacy, keep that in a separate place).

Track your life for at least thirty days. Notice the rhythm of your days without judgment. Many habit experts talk about how important it is to track our daily activities—and to acknowledge even incremental changes over time. In our case, we're not setting out to change something—just observing. When we have a punishing voice in our head that's so strong it needs to cut our own skin, we want to be careful about how and when we apply willpower to change habits. It's a tricky balance. So, at first, just watch to see which activities bring relief or joy.

Ask yourself, what is the one thing you *love* to do most? For me, that's writing. Although naps are a close second. Painting is fun too. Oh, but I love eating too. And being at the beach. Especially if I can read at the beach. Every day I savor something I love—whether it's a pet, an activity, my partner, or Nature. When I *give* love, I get it back tenfold.

For each day you did something you love, track those markers too.

If you're working with different parts of your interior, you might notice which of them like which activity and if some of those aggravate other parts. For example, when I let Hope dance around by herself, L gets embarrassed and tries to stop her. But when we create art, all three parts join in—it's their favorite thing to do together. Are there any activities that bring your internal family together?

Is there one practice that you can identify that is essential to your well-being? Meditation is the one thing I *have* to do no matter what—I need to check in with my parts, call everyone together, connect with a higher power, and tap into the universal field. That's followed closely by the need for eight hours of sleep. When I go to bed early enough, I don't wake up with that old sense of dread. On the other hand, I'm gentle with myself when I *don't* go to bed on time. That struggle—between trying to do the right thing and beating myself up when I don't—had to be dismantled. Now, I use an app to track all of my positive habits so I get to experience pride when I'm doing well, and encouragement when I falter. This process offers valuable information about what needs to be changed next (but only when I'm ready).

This practice can evolve into something more sophisticated that works for you. Somewhere along the path of recovery, we all have to learn to manage our routines and come up with daily protocols to keep ourselves healthy. Whatever we create will need to be constantly tweaked. You may want to share with your therapist or guide to give you an objective viewpoint, but no doctor, medication, or outside influence is going to fix us. They are only guides. Healing is slow, and it happens over a lifetime of choices. Only we can walk that path.

Advanced Exercise: Create a Series

This chapter has been about mapping, documenting, and tracking. Have you ever done any of that in your work? Have you written an autobiography or memoir that puts everything in chronological or thematic order? Have you incorporated numbers, words, or grids into your visual art? Are you willing to try it?

If you tend to create organic or abstract forms, try superimposing geometrics into a piece. Let your usual shapes move in and out of the structure. Or if you're already a geometric painter, add some abstraction. Create a piece (or series) that incorporates both approaches. Stay inquisitive while you work. What are the two modalities saying to one another? How does it feel to go outside your comfort zone?

I've recently started incorporating mandalas into my expressionist work. It started with wedges of geometrics that only barely contained the chaotic forms inside, then it progressed to full mandalas containing both abstract and realistic imagery. How can you add or subtract structure within your work? Does it give more meaning to what you've been doing?

Another idea is to explore the concept of maps within your work. It can be internal—creating a map of your own journey—or external, like a study of old maps and what it meant within the history of that time. You could map an abstraction, like the history of sadness, or document a concrete statistic within an unexpected form—like gridding out the number of species dying every year, laid out in the shape of a tree.

The conceptual artist Charles Gaines is a genius at this. He often utilizes natural forms in his work, combining imagery with numbered grids, in his critique of systems and representation. Whereas Gaines limits this exploration to intellectual realms as a way to challenge social and political systems, in our case, we're taking the structural form into emotional realms to contain internal chaos and learn more about ourselves.

Reflection

Before moving forward, take some time to journal about everything you learned at this stage. It's a lot to take in. These exercises are meant to start you on a path that you will take over for yourself.

Whether or not you develop your own protocol to maintain healing, the most important element is love. Loving yourself, loving the process, loving the unknown.

I share gratitude lists on an email chain with friends—and we also list one example of where we saw God. In other words, what amazing moment showed the beauty of Nature? What encounter revealed Spirit in another person? What synchronicity lit us up with wonder?

No matter how heavy my day is, something always reminds me how miraculous life is. Those of us who have survived horrors inside our own heads can appreciate the Light more than most.

Concluding Thoughts

Thus far, we've gone from passively experiencing our self-harming energy to drawing it out, engaging with it, naming it, giving it different tasks, and redirecting it in new ways. We identified fragmented parts inside—those experiential energies that are missing from terms like "dissociation" and "depersonalization." We're not empty—we're just cut off from vitality because of our responses to trauma. All of those pieces can be claimed and reassembled.

Creativity is the way in, the tool to sculpt our unique story.

This chapter focused on harnessing love. This tremendous spiritual force allows us to develop compassion for ourselves, to dig deeper into the work, and to connect to others. It's the healing salve that stitches up wounds.

Love reminds us that we have agency in our healing. We get to choose how fast we want to go, and what it looks like over time. We've always had that choice but didn't know it before. That's hard to remember when urges and parts overwhelm. But those come from inside *us*, not outside. Love allows us to *own* the parts we haven't wanted to accept before, and to integrate them into wholeness.

We also talked about the journey being its own destination. William Bridges, in his book *The Way of Transition*, said "…we achieve our breakthroughs not by setting out to break through, but by doing the work that is right in front of us."[21] He viewed his life experience through the lens of transition as an organizing narrative. What he discovered was that every journey is round-trip (it ends where it started), it exists at every level of our lives, and it is *being on the path*—the way—that changes us.

So, what happens next? All this tilling of the soil and planting seeds leads to what?

Those are the kinds of questions I've asked myself for years. It wasn't until I let go of having to know next steps that I could sense them ahead.

---

[21] William Bridges, *The Way of Transition: Embracing Life's Most Difficult Moments* (De Capo Press, 2001), 130.

"...it took me nearly a lifetime to learn to trust my heart."

—William Bridges

"When I stand before thee at the day's end, thou shalt see my scars and know that I had my wounds and also my healing."

—Rabindranath Tagore

CHAPTER EIGHT

ALLOWING GRACE

How do you know when you've turned a corner in recovery? I used to think that was when I started to feel better. But "feeling better" is an elusive state, and if I tie my sense of well-being to that state, I will remain confused and insecure. Because feelings are not facts—they're like clouds against the sky. I—that is, my true Self—I am the sky, not the cloud. It's vast and immutable, the backdrop for everything that happens within it.

However, one turning point that stood out was the point when I started to really care about others—to use my painful past and the tools it taught me to help those who were struggling. I had to be self-centered during those healing years. Once I got better, I *wanted* to help others.

Members of 12-step programs know that service to newcomers is a vital part of recovery, a spiritual necessity. That's what this book has been for me—a way to offer hope to others. If it can help people who self-injure find healing, or professionals working with self-harming clients, then it will be a success. Whatever happens from here is not up to me. I can only offer it up with my love and prayers.

Which brings me to the subject I've touched upon several times in this book—the role of Spirit, or God if you prefer, in the healing process.

I use the word God sometimes because it's easier, but in many circles, it activates security fences around peoples' belief systems. To me, the word represents more of a Creative Intelligence, the guiding force that propels all growth, all evolution. It's what heals my wounds. It's Love at its unconditional best. It's the bigger Self who observes my smaller ego self. It's the mystery behind everything. My Lady of Light is just my own version—something safe to attach to—the greater Whole is beyond my ability to describe.

Whatever it is to you, lean into it. If you're an atheist or agnostic, there's always the power of love, nature, or grace.

To me, grace is a state of being that produces miracles—not turning-water-into-wine type of miracles, but the kind that transcend what we can engineer on our own. Like healing from self-harming. Or getting sober from an addiction. The same intelligent forces that heal wounded skin also operate on a mental and spiritual level to form new pathways. All we have to do is start the work and get out of the way. New shoots know how to grow into full plants.

One of the by-products of being in Grace is forgiveness. David R. Hawkins said, "Forgiveness is an aspect of love that allows us to see life events from the viewpoint of grace."[22] But it can be a thorny subject—especially if there's been abuse and betrayal. We hold onto painful memories because they're familiar, and the familiar protects us from the unknown. I would never push anyone to forgive before they're ready—that's like peeling off a layer of new skin before it's healed. Besides, in my experience, true forgiveness is not a goal to

---

[22] Hawkins, *Letting Go*, 175.

be achieved through direct action—it's a gift of Grace, and it comes when we're ready, whether we think we are or not.

And its power is beyond compare.

My Experience

For me, healing has not been a one-and-done deal. It has come in overlapping circles, each one wider and deeper than the last. It will continue to cycle around as long as I'm alive. Because one day, I'll have to deal with the biggest loss of all—my own life on this planet and the body I've (finally) become attached to.

My first round came after my suicide attempt at seventeen, when I dropped some defenses and let Mrs. Hren help me. Her assistance got me to the next chapter, which began with a full scholarship and a ticket to my life in California.

The second came when I surrendered at twenty-four and admitted I was an alcoholic and addict. Once again, I let others in on my secrets. The change in my behaviors led to uncovering memories of being sexually abused. Reopening those wounds led to more healing, thanks to a lot of help from therapy, recovery, and friendships.

The third big cycle came when my father was dying. We'd been in contact for three years at that point, after seven years of silence. During that period, I'd written many angry letters that I never sent, but one day, forgiveness appeared in my heart. My brother's wedding was coming up and I didn't want my rift with our father to cause extra drama, so I called Dad. He was still in denial, so we agreed to disagree. The truth was I'd missed him. When I no longer needed him to admit what he'd done, I was able to be in a relationship with him again. He was still his inappropriate self, but every time he made a weird sex joke, I held up my hand and reminded him he was my father, and he laughed it off.

When we got the official word that his kidney tumor was inoperable and terminal, I went to visit him at his Florida "home"—which turned out to be a storage warehouse with a hospice cot installed in the front room, not the multi-disciplinary art colony he'd bragged about. He'd been living in his van for a long time, and now rented a warehouse on a dead-end lane. All his stuff was strewn about, and everything was riddled with cockroaches. He sold drugs to make the rent and pay for the five packs of cigarettes he smoked every day.

And yet I also witnessed how kind he was to his friends—society's outsiders like him. On my second visit two months later, I turned thirty-five and he bought me a book about cats—the only gift I'd gotten from him since my teenage years. That night, we sat on the beach and cried together. On my third and last visit, seeing his thin body so weakened by the cancer, the last of my anger drained away. Even with his confusing deathbed confession, I was done with anger. The morning I left, I whispered into his ear that I loved him, forgave him, and I'd carry his potential with me. I was finally able to see the many gifts he'd given me. Writing about him and our life together turned me into a writer. And forgiving him gave me strength I never knew I had.

The fourth round of healing came after my partner's parents died and our relationship fell apart, ending in divorce. Those losses plunged me into the depths of pain. The assumptions and beliefs I'd held for twenty years crumbled away, and I slid into darkness. But I wasn't alone. My therapist helped me through, and so did many friends who appeared by my side. I met the woman who would become my partner, and eventually, my wife. I finally mapped the terrain of my own abyss. I got to know Faith, Hope, and Love. I reclaimed the parts that had been frozen in time, freeing up vast reserves of energy to begin a new life. I found a partner in Spirit.

The fifth round also came through loss. I'd been trying to help my brother with his addictions for years. Part of me knew I was ineffective, but I kept trying anyway. When I finally let go of that with the help of another recovery program, I was able to have a loving relationship with him that was free of judgment. I'm so grateful for that time because his overdose at the end of 2021 destroyed much of his brain and wiped out the Andy we'd known. He lived for six miserable weeks until he finally succumbed to Covid. During this time, my mother and I let go of long-standing resentments and drew together.

After Andy died and I saw how the abuse had twisted him up inside, I got angry at Dad again—but it wasn't the same as before. The anger was grounded in compassion and matured by grief. Dad had done the best with what he had. So had Andy. How or why I got the strength to choose a different path is still a mystery to me—but I no longer use it to judge others who make different choices. I feel closer to Andy now than I have since we were kids—I know he's there and will greet me when I pass over. His daughters are beautiful examples of his spirit living on, and the experience brought me closer to them as well.

He also showed me how short and precious life is. I spent so much time trying to escape it when what I really wanted to escape was the pain. With Andy's death, I embraced it. I cared for myself and my body as I was going through the loss. I gave everything I had to help others in their grief. I let myself be overrun by waves, rubbed down by saltwater, abraded by tears.

I see more losses in my future, as I move beyond the steady fading of youth. My mother is getting older, pets I adore will pass away, and my partner may leave this planet before I do. My resistance falls away more every year—and what grows in its place is a steady acceptance of everything I cannot change. The only thing I can change is myself. I exert the strength and willpower I've gained from reclaiming my child parts to achieve goals, but the results are not up to me. I do the work and offer it up to God.

As you might have noticed by now, the theme that threads all these cycles together is *letting go*. Some might call it radical acceptance. William Bridges put it this way, "...life runs a perfect curriculum, and the tuition is modest...it offers us a correspondence course in letting go, Introductory Letting Go, Intermediate Letting Go, and Advanced Letting Go."[23] Knowing that gives me comfort. If I resist loss by gripping tighter, I suffer more—but when I sink deeper into it and surrender the outcome, the feelings pass through me, and I experience new growth.

Here's something else I noticed—during each cycle of healing, I found a deeper connection with a higher power. The closer I was to death, the more intense the experience. Lady of Light came to me after the suicide attempt. On the last night I drank and used drugs, I considered killing myself, but then I felt powerful wings around me, and I found the strength to call a friend in recovery. Doing yoga kept me connected to spiritual practices, even if I struggled with the word "God." I claimed to be atheist/agnostic for years—but after my divorce, I realized I did believe in something, and I needed to find out what that was. And so, I embarked on a search for it. I read, meditated, prayed, listened, wrote, and created art. It all came together during a yoga class one day, when I was deep into my work with my inner parts. I felt a stirring inside my body—inside *me*—that connected to what felt like God-energy. Lady of Light, the

---

[23] Bridges, *The Way of Transition*, 81.

dragon, and the tree were as real as ever—but they were only part of the larger Spirit in and around all things.

Another thing I realized was that I was never truly alone, even at my loneliest. People always appeared at the exact right time to give just what I needed. These teachers, friends, therapists, and helpers were all physical expressions of Spirit. By now, I trust that they will continue to show up as I need them.

As my friend Theresa used to say, "I wish God had skin." In my experience, God shows up in the form of other people. We all need someone to hold our hands when we cry or take us out to dinner when we're sad. Or guide us through the throes of trauma recovery. So, Love comes in forms we can recognize.

I learned that one of the best teachers is the experience of loss. Each time I lost someone or something dear to me, it led to gifts I didn't know were there. And each opened my heart to more love. When I was a kid, we had a quote on our refrigerator that said, "Grief is a miner, carving out new chambers of the heart for love to fill." Whenever I lose someone, or a pet dies, I think I won't ever heal from the sorrow—but then another person or animal comes along, and I love them even more.

The point of loving is not to keep the object of our love, but to love no matter what. It's a current that flows through us and out. It only fills us up if we give it away.

Each cycle of destruction led to new growth, new creativity, new life—not without grief and sorrow but with new resilience. I only know I can get through hard things once I've gotten through hard things.

There's a whole field of psychology devoted to the study of Post-Traumatic Growth or the ways in which trauma builds resiliency. Calhoun and Tedeschi first published their findings in

1996,[24] building upon previous work in the field by practitioners/ philosophers like Viktor Frankl, Abraham Maslow, Irvin Yalom, Morton Lieberman, and more. Donald Meichenbaum developed a Post Traumatic Growth Inventory (PTGI) to quantify the process.

Some consider their work controversial, because it can be interpreted as a hierarchical system that values those who can "get over it" sooner. Also, those who experience certain traumas, especially early and chronic sexual abuse, tend to score lower on the tests—but that's because of the damaging nature of the trauma, not the subjects' resiliency.

I've never taken the PTGI test or been evaluated by people in that field, but I know that I've learned great lessons from what I've gone through, and I can see that most when I share my experience with others. Service to others is the single most powerful tool to transform darkness into light. I can spend days or weeks inside my head, doing the work of healing, learning new insights, but it isn't until I help somebody else that the teachings solidify in my being.

I saw that clearly in the process of writing this book. It was reassuring to learn that many of the realizations that came to me organically are being confirmed by professionals in the fields of mental health and creativity, especially in Neuroarts and Internal Family Systems therapy. The research gave me more resources to share with others. As often happens, once I focused my energy and attention on using creativity to heal from self-harm, people started reaching out to me with exactly those dilemmas, asking for my help. It affirmed that I was on the right path.

It also gave my body of work the throughline I'd been looking for. I've used so many different styles and mediums in my creative

---

[24] Tedeschi RG, Calhoun LG. The Posttraumatic Growth Inventory: measuring the positive legacy of trauma. J Trauma Stress. 1996 Jul;9(3):455-71. doi: 10.1007/BF02103658. PMID: 8827649.

practice that it's been difficult to pinpoint what my work is about. But in tying it to the process of healing from self-harm, it all makes sense. Each creation stems from the desire to discover, integrate, and share with others. That's the voice on the skin of my art.

Most days now, my internal parts work together. They still retain some of their earlier innocence, but they're also maturing and evolving. They create *me* as we go along. We check in every morning after meditation. Each one shares what they're feeling, what they need. We agree to work together on the tasks of the day. The adult me appears as the "captain of the ship" who steers our vessel on its truest course, with the help of the best crew ever (Faith, Hope, and Love answer, *Aye, aye, captain!*). We call upon our spirit guides and thank God for all our gifts.

Sometime in 2023, I felt a strange sensation filling my solar plexus. It wasn't one of the parts. I sensed a tangle of black thread churning below my ribs. I observed it without judgment for a few weeks. Nothing much happened. It just sat there. Then one day during meditation, it unfurled into a field of energy that expanded outward and seamed itself together around me like a membrane. I asked its name, and without hesitation, I heard the word, *Grace*. I wondered if it was just a momentary experience; but it stuck around and grew stronger. It's there to this day. Sometimes it's a protective shield, sometimes it's a liquid body of energy. It doesn't have a distinct personality, so it's not a part. It just exists all around me.

I suppose it means I'm in a state of Grace.

I recently read this in a daily inspirational email: "What could be more valuable than peace of mind? With it, no other valuables are necessary. Without it, all the valuables in the world aren't enough."

And that's been true for me. It opens up a paradox that emerges alongside all the others, *I only get the things I'm seeking when I let go of wanting them.* I wanted freedom from pain, fulfilling relationships, financial security, and creative success—but once I accepted that they weren't the ultimate destination, I received them all. And I only keep them by letting them go, every day.

The only real goal is grace—which consists of love, hope, and faith. I'll never be free of pain and loss. No relationship can fill the hole inside me (and if it does, it's not healthy)—and no amount of money or success will bring me peace of mind. Once I accept my life just as it is—*amor fati*—I am content with what I have. I am enough.

Your Experience

This is the last chapter of teaching—but not the end of your learning. By now, if you've been doing the work, you will be on your own way to healing. The prompts in this book are just a beginning, a gate opening onto the path. Where it leads is unique to you.

The exercises below came out of a deeper connection, both within myself to Spirit, and with the world outside. I hope they inspire the same connections within you.

Grounding Technique: Cover Me

Just because we're healing doesn't mean we become immune to triggers. If our nervous systems were formed in an environment of trauma, we're hardwired to respond in certain ways, and it can take years of work to calm those down and change our automatic responses. It's important to keep employing grounding exercises.

One of my favorites is the simplest. I got it from a friend who served as a soldier during the Gulf War. When she encountered a dangerous situation, she'd say, "Cover me, God, I'm going in!"

And so, I (and many of our mutual friends) employ that same strategy. Whenever I'm afraid, or dealing with an overwhelming moment, I repeat those words. And I jump into the fray.

Visualization: The Family Together

This meditation involves another trip to your favorite place inside. Hopefully, by this stage, it has taken on more dimension and meaning and is easier to access. Start with whatever methods you've developed to relax into it—sit comfortably, wrap in a blanket, breathe deeply, etc. Drop into your environment. Settle into that familiarity, security, and anticipation.

Make your way to the Source, where your core Spirit dwells. Sit down with them. Take some time to breathe in the air, listen to sounds, and watch the movements of nature in your world. Feel the sacred energy here.

Beings are moving toward you. Soon, you see your teenager, your littlest one, the one who self-harmed, anyone else you've identified inside. Feel them gathering into one place, as if all the energy of the Universe is coalescing deep in your core. It swirls there, gently.

How do your parts greet each other? If it's only one child inside, how do they interact with your core spirit? Don't direct this play, just watch it. If there's any tension between parts, just observe it. Is there any new connection being made?

Notice if they come together in a specific place. Is there a tent, or shelter, or overhang, or temple? Are they sitting around a fire? Are they in a room? Let them show you where they like to gather, what they want to do together. Allow, observe, and explore. You have all the time in the world.

When you're ready, thank them for their courage, for being willing to meet each other. Acknowledge how hard each of them has worked to keep you intact. Appreciate their gifts. Tell them you look forward to seeing them again. Assure them that they can talk to you anytime they want.

Come out of the visualization with a deep breath and a big smile.

Journal what you observed. What does each part bring to the table? These are your gifts, and you can call upon them at any time. What does each part need? These are the areas that need work—not because you're deficient, but because you're a parent who is committed to providing for your kids.

Write about or sketch their gathering place. Name it with something you can remember easily, like *the tent*, or *the table*. That way, the next time you go inward to communicate with your parts, you can call them to the gathering place.

This is only the beginning of a lifetime of internal dialogue. Nothing is set in stone. It's been my experience that the landscape changes, the parts evolve, and the connections develop. This is the actual experience of what is happening when new neural pathways are forged in the brain—our interior narrative grows.

Exercise: The Tree of Me

The next exercise involves a tree again—but this time, you'll be creating "the tree of me."

Tune into your body, call upon the child parts, summon them to the gathering place. Tell them you'd like their help to create a fun illustration that will require all of their contributions. Each one will get equal time.

In your journal or on a sheet of paper, draw a rough shape of a trunk and a crown. Draw a line to represent the ground it sits on, then sketch out some roots below.

Now, with the help of your inner kids, place each part of you somewhere in the trunk. They may be in different places or nested inside each other. This is the body of your mind—the place where your psyche dwells. What does that feel like, and how can you represent that in a drawing? Do images of animals come to you? If you're uncomfortable drawing, can you write words inside that tree and let them represent the parts of you? What about using different colors for each one?

Draw or write the kids' concepts of Spirit. Is it inside the trunk or outside? Is it in the crown or the roots?

When you work on the roots, think about what shaped who you are. Draw or write your parents' contribution, your ancestors, your culture—acknowledge the illnesses and traumas, the gifts and good fortune. Does your concept of a higher power (or lack thereof) begin here? Connect those lines up through the trunk.

Bring branches up from the trunk into the crown. This is what you give to the world. What are the branches made of? Your work, your children, your recovery? Your spiritual beliefs? What connects you to others? What are you reaching for? Feel free to embellish with birds, nests, bugs, knots in the bark, hidden treasures—whatever comes to mind. Or just keep it a plain shape filled with words. It can be an oak, a fir, a palm, or whatever shape you prefer. It doesn't have to be perfect. The crown may change with the seasons, but the roots and trunk are solid—they are the essence of you. Pay attention to what that contains.

Return to the illustration whenever you want to add something. It's growing just as you are. Let it teach you things you hadn't realized before. You are as connected to the earth and sky as any living thing. Your story began long before you were born, and your gifts will reverberate long after you're gone (whether you know it or not). See yourself placed firmly in this forest of humanity. You have a valuable place in it and a right to thrive and contribute.

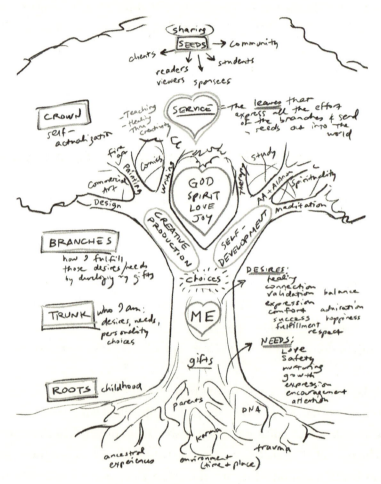

Figure 13: "The Tree of Me," 2020, one of many attempts to map out my interior in a way that made sense.

Exercise: An Autobiography

In one of my recovery programs, we have newcomers write an autobiography—not a novel-length memoir, but a story in broad strokes, like an extended essay. I found it to be a powerful tool.

The important thing is to start from the beginning, whatever that means—either your birth, or how your parents met, or the cultural milieu you were born into. Write it as a first-person narrative. Don't worry about length or content. It will have a beginning, middle, and end, but with room for new chapters.

You might want to revisit your map. Look for trends in the types of transitions you went through. Could you divide it into chapters? And if so, what would you title them? What would you title the book? Is there a clear theme throughout the book or chapter, like Learning Through Loss, or Triumphing over Adversity?

If you had to describe it in an elevator pitch, what sentence or phrase would encompass the whole thing? What would the deep-voiced movie announcer say about it in a trailer? What's the open-ended hook that leaves viewers guessing?

For example, my movie trailer might say, "An artist who has spent her entire life trying to escape the ravages of trauma and self-harming finally finds a way out, and shares what she learned with the world. Can she get her message out in time?"

A little bit of humor goes a long way.

Exercise: Art with Grace

This one's a little different. Instead of exploring your interior, you're going to make a gift for someone else.

First, decide on what you'd like to create that will embody love and connection. You might paint a message on a rock or draw on the front of a greeting card. You could sculpt a heart, or an angel, or a funny creature. You could color a mandala.

Next, choose someone to give it to. It could be a friend in need. Or maybe a person who is living on the street—in which case, you might add a little money, or a pair of socks. Think about what would brighten their world.

But before you give it to them, there's a catch. It has to be anonymous. You can't tell anyone about it, even your partner or therapist. No one. (KC suggested this exercise once, and it was a profound experience for me.)

How does anonymity change what you'll create? What will you write? Can you be even more loving in your message when no one knows it's you?

This is not about getting credit for being a good person—this is another way to connect with the flow of Spirit. If the sages are right and we're all One, then you're offering love to yourself. Let go of the small self and love the greater Self.

Advanced Exercise: The Communal

Use your medium of choice to depict your true family—the ancestral and cultural tree that preceded your birth, the structure of your internal parts, and your place in the human forest. You might include your family or origin, you might not. See if you can stretch a little. Incorporate another medium into your work or increase the scale.

I prefer to work on small to medium-size canvases because of the limitations of my studio, but once I painted a 5-by-8-foot piece to depict a larger story of me and how I relate to the "grand and damaging parade." It included a self-portrait with three faces, all the cats I took care of at the time, my father as an archetypal wanderer, images of my childhood, a transgender angel, and names of people who had supported me carved into the background.

If you've never painted a mural before, this is the perfect time to try it. If you can't find a free wall, you can paint on a large plywood panel. But don't do it alone—enlist help from loved ones, like I did with my mandala murals. If you design the template, all they have to do is fill in colors. Pick your own imagery that creates community and a process that brings everyone together. People love having the opportunity to paint without feeling judged. Let creativity unite you into a family.

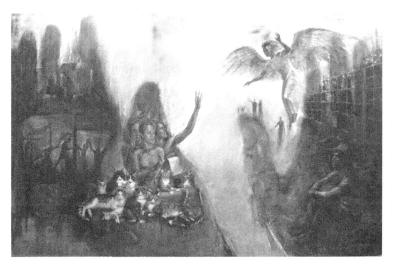

Figure 14: "The Grand and Damaging Parade," Oil on canvas, 2005-2008. Inspired by Kay Ryan's poetry.

Reflection

As you journal about the insights from this chapter, note the tone of your writing. Go back and review earlier entries. Is there a difference? Can you see a shift?

The process of becoming whole is gradual, and it moves in fits and starts. But somewhere along the way, corners are turned. Blinders fall away and we can see things more clearly. We never reach a plateau that's free of challenges and pain, but that old feeling of dread diminishes and eventually disappears.

I promise it does.

I probably should have warned you in the beginning, but once you start the process of healing, you can't go back. Of course, you can try to hold on to what's familiar—but it gets harder and harder.

During one of my last self-harming sessions, toward the end of my healing process, I found that it had already changed. It actually *hurt* for the first time. It was like trying on an old outfit that no longer fit. By this time, I knew too much about what the cutting meant. Faith needed to be heard, L had to numb the skin, Hope had to go to sleep—but once I understood the full dynamic, it no longer worked.

So, I had no choice but to put the blade down. I had to re-commit to my pilgrimage of healing. The only way around it was *through* it—and as I progressed, my escape routes began to disappear behind me.

What escape routes have closed behind you? What are you no longer willing to do, to tolerate, to experience in your own life? What rituals and behaviors are now essential to your well-being?

What is your concept of God/Spirit? How has that changed over the course of this book? What does Grace mean to you?

Concluding Thoughts

This chapter has been about new beginnings, and the open-ended nature of healing. It's also about Spirit, and Creativity in its greater form—the organic force of destruction and building anew that operates throughout our lives. When we engage in the art-making process, no matter our skills, we are tapping into this greater energy. Just like parents, whatever we bring into this world will have its own life. We need to trust where it's leading us.

The path of healing is cyclical, not linear. Rather than thinking of it as an endless loop, we might see it as circling deeper inward to the truth we've been looking for. And even then, there's more to learn. Nature is constantly evolving. Even if it's moving toward destruction, that's because it's preparing to re-emerge as something new.

But what about climate change, the destruction of the natural world, the collapse of societies, and evil? Those are the questions that used to discourage me from even trying. What's the point if it all ends in an ash heap?

We humans think we're the be-all and end-all of existence—but we're actually just one form of consciousness on a tiny planet circling one of billions of stars throughout the universe. Every ounce of pain I've felt in my life is just a microscopic speck in the scheme of things.

And yet.

That feeling I get when I paint something from the truth of me, when I see a perfectly round sphere of dew on the neighbor's mulberry tree, when I look into my dog's eyes, or when love pours through me to someone else…these are the things that make life worth living. As Camus said, "There is no love of life without despair of life."[25] Being able to hold both in our hearts without having to favor one or the other is a mark of true maturity.

After so many years of trying to escape the pain, when I turned around to face and embrace it, I found not only myself, but the

---

[25] Albert Camus, *Lyrical, and Critical Essays* (Vintage Books, 1970, Kindle Edition), 56.

Spirit I'd been searching for all along. Once I found it, the outside things didn't matter as much—or more specifically, they mattered in a *deeper* way. I realized I can't hold onto anything. Only Spirit endures, the true state of being beneath and inside the material world.

Something bigger is at work here—something that can only be accessed through creative and spiritual means. Psychology can offer crucial insights and guidance, and medicine can balance chemistry and aid in healing. But as important as those fields are, they are not equipped to provide us with the most important aspects of all—the willingness to change, to do the work, to enlist the help of Spirit.

These aspects are ours alone to claim.

"The passage of a life should show; it should abrade. And when life stops, a certain space—however small—should be left scarred by the grand and damaging parade. Things shouldn't be so hard."

—Kay Ryan, from her poem, *Things Shouldn't Be So Hard*

"The most beautiful people we have known are those who have known defeat, known suffering, known struggle, known loss, and have found their way out of the depths. These persons have an appreciation, a sensitivity, and an understanding of life that fills them with compassion, gentleness, and a deep loving concern. Beautiful people do not just happen."

—Elisabeth Kübler-Ross

CHAPTER NINE

BACK TO THE BEGINNING

And so, we come to the end of this guidebook. Perhaps it felt like a lot to take in. These aren't simple art games to be done mindlessly in front of the TV—they're deep-sea dives into your own psyche. Once you open the door, more pathways open up, and the story starts to create itself. The layers of the onion peel away, revealing deeper and deeper layers of yourself.

I've found that the further I progress in my healing, the more I keep finding myself back at the beginning—not only back to my youngest self, the beginning of me, but also to the same lessons in different forms. It's a paradox that can be seen from many different angles, like a prism.

You probably noticed that I listed a spiritual paradox in each chapter. These insights emerged as I was writing this book—not as forced conclusions, but as organic realizations that had been there all along.

I'll reiterate them here:

> *The wound holds the answer.*

> *The trauma creates the tools we need to heal from it.*

We have to ask the one who doesn't trust to have faith.

The only way around the problem is to go right through it.

We become stronger by being more vulnerable, not less.

The journey is the destination. We only get the things we're seeking when we let go of wanting them.

We are material and spiritual at the same time.

These truisms aren't just mystical, they're confirmed in the physical world as well. Quantum physics has proven that matter can exist as both a wave and a particle at the same time. Buffalos lean into the storm to get through it faster. We build muscle strength by tearing down existing tissue so that more of it grows back. When a broken bone heals, that site is stronger than it was before. We cut back trees and flowers to encourage growth.

A wound knows how to heal itself.

The hero's journey is not from one place to another, it's a full-circle return. The point is not to become someone else, it's to learn something valuable about our interior that can be shared with others.

Applying this to the dilemma posed by self-harming behaviors, we find that the act itself holds the key to what we seek. We must ask what the wound is trying to say. By pursuing the question, circling deeper and deeper, we finally discover the answer inside ourselves, where it was waiting for us to find it.

And creativity is the way in. As I've said, it's our birthright. We are creative, curious, problem-solving beings determined to evolve.

Those of us who have self-harmed are courageous. We're good at thinking outside the box. The behavior that hurt us can be turned into a valuable tool to help us and others.

All it takes is willingness, hard work, and time.

And Faith, Hope, Love, and Grace.

Final Thoughts

If you're like me, and you devoured this book like a bag of chips without stopping to do all the exercises, I hope you'll return to them when it feels right. And for those of you who skipped around or only did the exercises that called to you, that's okay too. It's not a linear path. You might find that you reach a plateau and wish to rest for a while, simply enjoying life. Then something happens to plunge you into deep feelings again. Keep the paradoxes in mind. Remember, my own process took decades to traverse, and it's still unfolding—yours will proceed at whatever pace is meant for you.

Every life has its sorrows—there's no escaping great pain. But if you've plumbed the depths of your own pain to find its source, you've discovered a rich vein that will yield unlimited truth, art, and compassion. It's the most authentic core of you—the connection to the greater Self that was lost through trauma.

I used to have over fifty scars on my body, from my forehead all the way down to my ankles. I once carved the words "I Want to Die" on my stomach, facing outwards for others to read. Over time, it faded so that all you could see was "I Want." That's mostly gone, too. The deepest scars on my inner arms are now obscured by tattoos. I no longer need to display the evidence to prove "it did happen." I believe Faith, Hope, and Love. They know they can get what they need from me, and our internal dialog continues to grow and flourish.

My life today, although far from perfect, is pretty damn good. I've finally found that thing I was seeking all along—internal peace and self-love. That's reflected outwardly in my marriage and in my relationships with family and friends. Forgiveness has deepened. I appreciate my mother more with every passing year. She's given me so many gifts, including the example of how to age gracefully.

I've tried to share as much of my experience as I could to help you navigate your own waters—but the details of your journey are yours to create.

Everyone has to find their own balance of self-care amidst the challenges of life. No one escapes without losing what's most important to them somewhere along the way. It's how we become real, as the velveteen rabbit taught us. The wound is where the light comes in—it's also where our love pours out.

I wish you peace and joy. Thank you for trusting me to guide you on a new path. I can't wait to see what you create next.

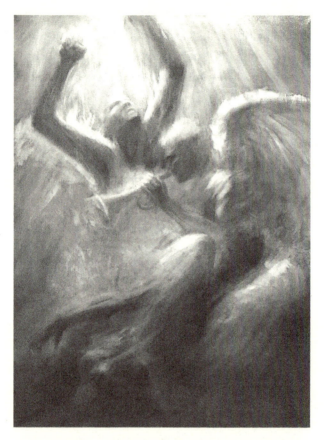

Figure 15: "Sea of Light," Oil on canvas, 2016. Someone once asked me about my paintings, "Maggie, where are they all going?" Hopefully, somewhere good.

ACKNOWLEDGEMENTS

I am deeply grateful for the kindness, support, guidance, and insight I received from so many people on the journey to publishing this book.

Thank you to Christine Bagni at Wandering Words Media for being the first to offer praise and constructive comments on the manuscript and to Sandra Wissinger for bringing it home. And to my early readers—Liz Koskenmaki, Angel Slimocosky, and Barbara Hancock, M.A., LMFT—your feedback was crucial to shaping my rough draft into a polished book. My friendships with you buoy me up. My mother read the manuscript in two days and gave me the approval I needed to move forward. Mom, you continue to amaze me with your grace, love, and courage in facing the things that most parents avoid.

I am eternally grateful to Jo Christner, Psy.D., for unwavering support and masterful guidance leading me from darkness into light. I could not have done this work without you, Dr. Jo.

My fellows in recovery, although anonymous, are my rock and my wings. Thank you for this day, which is all we really have.

And without a supportive partner, I could not have spent so much of my time and income on what has always been a labor of love. Thank you, Marylou, for everything. Your dedication to service inspires me every day.

ABOUT MAGGIE PARR

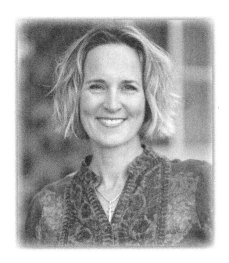

Maggie Parr is an artist and author who has designed theme park attractions, painted murals and portraits, and written and illustrated books and comics. She holds a Masters of Fine Arts (MFA), maintains a painting practice and teaches classical oil painting techniques to students from all backgrounds.

Expressionist artmaking helped her recover from decades of self-harming. As a result, she now mentors other creatives in their journeys to break through blocks and heal from trauma.

To learn more about the author or the concepts in this book, visit www.maggieparr.com or www.stoppingselfharm.com.

LAST WORDS

If you resonated with the concepts in this book, if it helped you in any way, please share it with others who might benefit as well. And should you feel moved to leave a positive review on Amazon, I would be most grateful!

And finally, if you would like to dive deeper into the work, visit www.stoppingselfharm.com to explore options. There, you can download free resources, take an online course, sign up for a workshop, work with me one-on-one, or just send me an email. I would love to hear about how this book has helped in your healing, and to see what you created in response to these exercises.

May you find your way back into wholeness. With love and light,

Maggie Parr

Made in United States
Orlando, FL
23 June 2025